Super Easy Diabetic Food Bible

The Ultimate Guide with 365+ Days of Low-GI, Low-Carb & Low-Sugar Recipes | 60-Day Meal Plan to Balance Blood Sugar, Manage Prediabetes, and Control Type 2 Diabetes

Without Giving Up the Foods You Love

Andrew Moore

Copyright © 2025 By Andrew Moore. All rights reserved.

No part of this book may be reproduced, transmitted, or distributed in any form or by any means without permission in writing from the publisher, except in the case of brief quotations embodied in critical articles or reviews.

Legal & Disclaimer

The content and information contained in this book has been compiled from reliable sources, which are accurate based on the knowledge, belief, expertise and information of the Author. The author cannot be held liable for any omissions and/or errors.

TABLE OF CONTENTS

EDITOR'S LETTER 10
   Why This Cookbook Stands Out 10

CHAPTER 1: GETTING STARTED — THE ESSENTIALS OF DIABETES & HEALTHY EATING 10
   Understanding the Types of Diabetes 11
   Why Diabetes Happens: Getting to the Root .. 11
   Eating Made Simple: What to Choose for Better Blood Sugar 12
   Must-Know Nutrition Tips: Reading Labels That Matter 12
   Ingredients to Limit or Avoid for Better Blood Sugar 13
   Smart Ingredient Picks for Diabetic-Friendly Meals 14
   Simple Kitchen Tips to Keep Blood Sugar Balanced 14

CHAPTER 2: 60-DAY MEAL PLAN 16

CHAPTER 3: BREAKFAST: Quick and Easy Diabetic-Friendly Breakfast Ideas 20
   Turkey Sausage and Veggie Scramble 21
   Hard-Boiled Eggs with Avocado and Spinach Salad 21
   Cottage Cheese with Fresh Peaches and a Drizzle of Honey 21
   Apple Cinnamon Overnight Oats with Flaxseeds 22
   Chia Seed Pudding with Coconut Milk and Raspberries 22
   Greek Yogurt Parfait with Walnuts and Mixed Berries 22
   Spinach and Feta Scramble with a Side of Sautéed Mushrooms 23
   Asparagus and Goat Cheese Omelette with Fresh Herbs 23
   Sautéed Zucchini and Bell Pepper Frittata 23
   Egg Muffins with Bell Peppers and Spinach. 24
   Almond-Crusted Zucchini Fritters with Poached Eggs 24
   Warm Kale and Quinoa Breakfast Bowl with Soft-Boiled Egg 24
   Savory Quinoa Breakfast Bowl 25
   Cottage Cheese and Walnut Toast 25
   Spinach and Mushroom Egg Muffins 25
   Zucchini and Feta Omelet 26
   Avocado and Tofu Breakfast Bowl 26
   Sweet Potato and Spinach Hash with Egg 26
   Tofu Scramble with Peppers and Spinach 27
   Berry Almond Quinoa Bowl 27
   Turkey and Veggie Breakfast Patties 27

Low-Carb Breakfast Bowls and Smoothies 28
   Creamy Avocado and Spinach Smoothie Bowl with Chia Seeds 28
   Green Keto Smoothie with Coconut Milk and Almond Butter 28
   Cucumber and Kale Smoothie 28
   Pumpkin and Cinnamon Smoothie 29
   Cinnamon Quinoa Breakfast Bowl with Almonds and Berries 29
   Chia and Flax Seed Porridge with Coconut Milk and Blueberries 29
   Pumpkin Spice Quinoa Porridge with Almond Milk 30
   Flaxseed Porridge with Cinnamon and Chopped Pecans 30
   Buckwheat Porridge with Almonds and Raspberries 30
   Almond Butter Couscous Porridge with Blueberries and Flaxseeds 31
   Kale and Coconut Protein Bowl 31
   Blueberry Spinach Smoothie with Flaxseeds 31
   Savory Greek Bowl with Eggs and Olives. 32
   Avocado and Chia Seed Smoothie 32
   Zucchini and Egg Protein Bowl 32
   Strawberry Almond Breakfast Smoothie ... 33
   Cauliflower and Egg Power Bowl 33
   Nutty Green Smoothie with Zucchini and Almonds 33

High-Protein Dishes to Stabilize Blood Sugar. 34
   Broccoli and Cheddar Scramble with Herbs. 34
   Soft-Boiled Eggs with Sautéed Kale and Mushrooms 34
   Spinach and Feta Stuffed Chicken Breasts.. 34

- Egg White and Turkey Sausage Scramble... 35
- Grilled Chicken Salad with Avocado and Quinoa..35
- Beef and Broccoli Stir-Fry with Sesame Seeds...35
- Turkey and Spinach Meatballs with Zucchini Noodles..36
- Egg and Spinach Breakfast Muffins with Turkey Bacon...36
- Chicken and Chickpea Salad with Avocado and Lime.. 36
- Grilled Steak with Roasted Vegetables and Quinoa...37
- Turkey and Black Bean Chili with Avocado... 37
- Baked Chicken Thighs with Roasted Cauliflower.. 37
- Low-Carb Cottage Cheese and Spinach Pancakes.. 38
- Lentil and Quinoa Stew with Turkey Sausage...38
- Turkey Lettuce Wraps with Avocado and Cucumber..38
- Grilled Chicken Bowl with Spinach and Tahini..39
- Lentil and Turkey Mini Patties...................39
- Egg and Cottage Cheese Bake with Broccoli.. 39
- Beef and Zucchini Skillet...........................40
- Baked Tofu Nuggets with Mustard Dip......40
- Egg, Kale and Turkey Stir-Fry...................40
- Cottage Cheese Omelet with Herbs..........41
- Turkey and Cabbage Stir-Fry.....................41
- Tuna Salad Bowl with Boiled Egg and Greens.. 41

Weekend Brunch Ideas................................ 42
- Crustless Veggie Quiche with Bell Peppers and Onions..42
- Zucchini and Egg Casserole with Feta and Oregano.. 42
- Mushroom and Asparagus Egg Bake....... 42
- Cauliflower Rice Stir-Fry with Scrambled Eggs and Garlic.......................................43
- Almond Flour Pancakes with Blueberry Compote..43
- Coconut Flour Waffles with Cinnamon and Almond Butter.......................................43
- Keto Pumpkin Pancakes with Pecans.......44
- Low-Carb Zucchini Fritters with Poached Eggs.. 44
- Almond Flour Crepes with Ricotta and Spinach.. 44
- Low-Carb Pizzas with Turkey and Spinach... 45
- Eggplant Breakfast Pizza with Scrambled Eggs and Parmesan.................................45
- Buckwheat Pancakes with Cinnamon and Walnuts.. 45
- Crustless Quiche with Spinach, Mushrooms, and Feta.. 46
- Baked Zucchini Turkey Fritters..................46
- Coconut Yogurt Parfait with Berries and Seeds.. 46
- Egg-Stuffed Bell Pepper Boats................. 47
- Mini Broccoli and Cheese Casserole......... 47
- Warm Chia Almond Porridge with Berries. 47
- Eggplant and Goat Cheese Stack............. 48
- Turkey, Arugula & Avocado Lettuce Wraps... 48
- Stuffed Portobello Mushrooms with Egg... 48

CHAPTER 4: LUNCH: Hearty Soups and Stews for Balanced Blood Sugar................................49
- Beef and Vegetable Stew with Carrots and Celery..49
- Creamy Cauliflower and Leek Soup with Roasted Garlic..................................... 49
- Creamy Broccoli and Cauliflower Soup with Almonds.. 49
- Chicken and Quinoa Soup with Spinach and Herbs..50
- Chicken and Lentil Stew............................50
- Butternut Squash and Turkey Chili............50
- Beef and Barley Soup with Root Vegetables 51
- Turkey and White Bean Soup with Fresh Cilantro..51
- Vegetable and Ground Beef Stew with Zucchini..51
- Savory Beef and Mushroom Stew with Fresh Thyme.......................................52
- Root Vegetable and Beef Stew with Fresh Parsley.. 52
- Creamy Mushroom Soup with Roasted

Garlic and Herbs 52
Tomato and Red Lentil Soup with Fresh Basil 53
Green Vegetable Stew with Chicken and Dill 53
Egg Drop Soup with Mushrooms and Bok Choy 53
Turkey and Spinach Soup with Lemon 54
Cabbage and Beef Tomato Stew 54
Creamy Turnip and Leek Soup 54
Eggplant Chickpea Stew with Tahini 55
Garlic Turkey Meatball Soup with Greens . 55
Zucchini and Herb Soup with Poached Egg .. 55

Low-Glycemic Grain Bowls 56

Bulgur Wheat Bowl with Ground Turkey and Zucchini 56
Millet and Carrot Bowl with Turkey Meatballs 56
Farro and Grilled Vegetables with a Yogurt-Tahini Dressing 56
Quinoa Bowl with Grilled Chicken and Roasted Peppers 57
Barley and Mushroom Bowl with Baby Kale. 57
Buckwheat and Roasted Broccoli Bowl with Sunflower Seeds 57
Quinoa and Roasted Veggie Bowl with Tahini Dressing 58
Buckwheat Bowl with Grilled Chicken and Avocado 58
Millet and Roasted Cauliflower Bowl with Lemon Vinaigrette 58
Barley and Roasted Red Pepper Bowl with Turkey 59
Quinoa with Sautéed Spinach and Avocado. 59
Farro Bowl with Roasted Butternut Squash and Chicken 59
Freekeh Bowl with Roasted Brussels Sprouts and Tahini Drizzle 60
Quinoa Bowl with Sautéed Swiss Chard and Poached Egg 60
Amaranth and Mushroom Bowl with Herb Yogurt Sauce 60
Teff Bowl with Roasted Carrot and Chickpeas 61
Barley Bowl with Grilled Tofu and Red Cabbage 61
Buckwheat Bowl with Smoked Salmon and Avocado 61
Quinoa and Black Bean Bowl with Cilantro-Lime Yogurt 62
Barley Bowl with Roasted Fennel and Chicken 62
Spelt Bowl with Sautéed Kale and Poached Egg 62

Wholesome Casseroles for Lasting Energy 63

Zucchini Lasagna with Ground Turkey and Ricotta 63
Eggplant Moussaka with Ground Beef and Parmesan 63
Spinach and Feta Crustless Quiche with Almond Flour 63
Chicken and Cauliflower Rice Casserole with Broccoli 64
Zucchini and Mushroom Lasagna with Ricotta and Mozzarella 64
Ground Turkey and Kale Casserole with Almond Crust 64
Mushroom and Ground Beef Casserole with Cauliflower 65
Spaghetti Squash Casserole with Chicken and Alfredo Sauce 65
Butternut Squash and Zucchini Lasagna with Turkey and Ricotta 65
Italian-Style Stuffed Zucchini Boats with Ricotta and Spinach 66
Spiced Ground Beef Stuffed Eggplants with Almonds and Herbs 66
Zucchini and Mushroom Stir-Fry with Garlic and Almonds 66
Broccoli and Turkey Breakfast Bake with Cheddar 67
Eggplant & Chicken Casserole with Herb Yogurt 67
Cabbage and Tofu Bake with Almond Crumble 67
Cauliflower and Sardine Casserole with Lemon-Parsley Crust 68
Tofu and Mushroom Crustless Pie with Herbs 68
Chard and Ricotta Bake with Tomato Slices. 68
Crustless Zucchini Pie with Goat Cheese and Dill 69

Baked Cabbage and Ground Beef Gratin with Cheese 69
Brussels Sprouts and Chicken Casserole with Almond Crust 69

Protein-Packed Meat Dishes 70
French-Style Baked Meat 70
Grilled Turkey Tenderloin with Roasted Vegetables 70
Stuffed Turkey Roll with Spinach & Feta ... 70
Grilled Flank Steak with Quinoa and Roasted Brussels Sprouts 71
Spinach and Ricotta-Stuffed Chicken Roll with Cauliflower Mash 71
Balsamic Glazed Beef Tenderloin with Garlic Sautéed Kale 71
Chicken Roulade with Goat Cheese & Tomatoes 72
Grilled Sirloin with Cauli Rice & Asparagus .. 72
Turkey Meatloaf Roll with Mushrooms 72
Beef Roll with Spinach, Feta & Eggplant .. 73
Pork Loin with Apple & Sage 73
Chicken Roll with Pesto & Mozzarella 73
Herb-Marinated Chicken Wings with Cauliflower Mash 74
Buffalo Chicken Wings with Cucumber and Celery Salad 74
Low-Carb BBQ Chicken Drumsticks with Coleslaw and Avocado 74
Rosemary Veal Chops with Steamed Broccolini 75
Spiced Lamb Patties with Mint Yogurt and Grilled Eggplant 75
Paprika Pork Medallions with Warm Tomato-Olive Salsa 75
Chicken Thighs with Dijon-Caper Sauce ... 76
Stuffed Cabbage Leaves with Beef and Herbs 76
Crispy Baked Pork Cutlets with Warm Fennel Slaw 76
Seared Duck Breast with Red Cabbage and Caraway 77
Beef & Spinach Skillet with Cherry Tomatoes 77
Baked Chicken Drumsticks with Veggie Sauté 77

CHAPTER 5: SNACKS AND DESSERTS:

Healthy, Low-Carb Snacks to Keep You Satisfied 78
Cucumber Slices with Avocado and Hummus 78
Stuffed Mini Bell Peppers with Cream Cheese and Herbs 78
Bell Pepper Strips with Guacamole 78
Spinach and Ricotta Stuffed Mushrooms .. 79
Cauliflower in Cheese Batter 79
Kale and Spinach Hummus with Almond Flour Crackers 79
Beetroot Hummus with Carrot and Zucchini Ribbons 80
Pumpkin Hummus with Cucumber 80
Olive and Sun-Dried Tomato Hummus with Zucchini 80
Deviled Eggs with Smoked Salmon and Avocado Mousse 81
Cilantro Lime Hummus with Bell Pepper Strips 81
Low-Carb Whole Grain Pita with Basil Pesto and Feta 81
Avocado Tuna Boats 82
Zucchini Chips with Parmesan Dust 82
Celery Sticks with Almond Butter and Chia Seeds 82
Smoked Salmon Rolls with Cucumber and Cream Cheese 83
Mini Eggplant Rounds with Herbed Goat Cheese 83
Hard-Boiled Eggs with Olive Tapenade 83
Stuffed Cherry Tomatoes with Avocado and Tuna 84
Cottage Cheese with Walnuts and Cinnamon 84
Radish Slices with Herbed Cream Cheese ... 84

High-Protein Options to Curb Cravings 85
Cottage Cheese with Sliced Tomatoes and Cucumber 85
Turkey and Cheese Skewers with Olives .. 85
Sliced Chicken Breast with Guacamole and Veggies 85
Tuna-Stuffed Avocados with Olive Oil and Lemon 86
Turkey and Avocado Lettuce Wraps 86
Hard-Boiled Eggs with Cottage Cheese and

Spinach... 86
Tuna Salad Lettuce Cups with Olive Oil....87
Chicken Salad with Avocado and Chia Seeds... 87
Spinach Egg Bites with Cottage Cheese.. 87
Chicken & Avocado Pita Wedges.............. 88
Ricotta-Stuffed Sweet Mini Peppers......... 88
Turkey and Cucumber Roll-Ups with Mustard Dip... 88
Tofu Salad with Greens and Lemon-Oil Dressing.. 89
Egg and Veggie Cups with Bell Pepper and Onion... 89
Avocado & Egg Mash on Zucchini Rounds... 89

Low-Sugar Dessert Recipes That Don't Spike Blood Sugar 90

Almond Flour Brownies with Dark Chocolate 90
Coconut Chia Pudding with Berries.......... 90
Sugar-Free Lemon Cheesecake Bites...... 90
Low-Sugar Chocolate Avocado Mousse... 91
Keto-Friendly Berry Cheesecake Bars...... 91
Sugar-Free Almond Butter Cups............. 91
Keto Pumpkin Pie Bites with Coconut Cream... 92
Cinnamon Almond Butter Cookies........... 92
Keto Lemon Bars with Coconut Crust....... 92
Lemon Poppy Seed Muffins with Almond Flour... 93
Strawberry and Coconut Cream Chia Parfait 93
Keto Chocolate Lava Cake with Dark Chocolate Filling..................................... 93
Almond Flour Snickerdoodle Cookies....... 94
Coconut Matcha Energy Balls.................. 94
Sugar-Free Raspberry Mousse with Whipped Coconut Cream........................ 94
Banana Nut Oat Bars with Almond Butter. 95
Blueberry Almond Mug Cake.................... 95
Cacao Coconut Bites with Allulose........... 95
Mini Lemon Ricotta Cups with Coconut Crust... 96
Strawberry Coconut Yogurt Bark.............. 96
Banana Almond Mug Muffin..................... 96
No-Bake Coconut Almond Bars................ 97

Cinnamon Vanilla Chia Custard................ 97
Hazelnut Cocoa Energy Truffles.............. 97

Delicious Cookies, Cakes, and Treats That Fit into Your Diabetic Plan 98

Coconut Flour Chocolate Chip Cookies.... 98
Almond Flour Lemon Poppy Seed Muffins 98
Keto Blueberry Mug Cake with Almond Flour... 98
Low-Sugar Apple Spice Cake with Almond Flour... 99
Sugar-Free Pumpkin Spice Cupcakes with Cream Cheese Frosting........................... 99
Low-Carb Chocolate Coconut Cookies..... 99
Coconut Flour Banana Bread with Chia Seeds.. 100
Almond Flour Peanut Butter Cookies......100
Keto-Friendly Lemon Coconut Cake....... 100
Cinnamon and Almond Keto Cupcakes.. 101
Low-Sugar Chocolate Almond Bars........ 101
Almond Flour Cinnamon Rolls with Cream Cheese Icing... 101
Keto Maple Pecan Scones...................... 102
Low-Sugar Apple Cinnamon Strudel with Almond Flour Crust............................... 102
Avocado and Almond Flour Matcha Cake with Creamy Lime Glaze........................ 102
Almond Coconut Ice Cream Bites........... 103
Orange Almond Biscotti.......................... 103
Vanilla Coconut Mini Donuts................... 103
Low-Carb Strawberry Shortcake Cups....104
Mini Chocolate Hazelnut Cakes.............. 104
Coconut Raspberry Thumbprint Cookies 104
Chocolate Zucchini Muffins with Almond Flour... 105
Mini Almond Butter Blondies................... 105
Coconut Flour Vanilla Cupcakes with Greek Yogurt Frosting..................................... 105

CHAPTER 6: DINNERS: Creative Salads with Diabetic-Friendly Dressings 106

Kale and Spinach Salad with Balsamic Vinaigrette and Feta............................... 106
Zucchini Noodle Salad with Pesto and Toasted Almonds.................................. 106
Arugula and Grilled Shrimp Salad with Citrus Dressing..................................... 106
Cauliflower Tabbouleh with Mint and Lemon Vinaigrette.. 107

Greek Salad with Grilled Halloumi and Olive Oil Dressing..................107
Cucumber and Radish Salad with Creamy Dill Yogurt Dressing..................107
Grilled Turkey and Mixed Greens Salad with Mustard Vinaigrette..................108
Spinach and Strawberry Salad with Poppy Seed Dressing..................108
Roasted Beet and Goat Cheese Salad with Balsamic Glaze..................108
Roasted Eggplant Salad with Tahini-Lemon Dressing..................109
Broccoli and Chickpea Salad with Garlic Yogurt Dressing..................109
Asian-Inspired Cabbage Salad with Sesame Ginger Dressing..................109
Avocado and Cucumber Salad with Lime-Cilantro Dressing..................110
Roasted Cauliflower and Chickpea Salad with Tahini-Garlic Dressing..................110
Spinach and Avocado Salad with Warm Mushroom Vinaigrette..................110
Grilled Eggplant Salad with Yogurt-Tahini Dressing..................111
Broccoli and Avocado Salad with Lemon-Garlic Dressing..................111
Red Cabbage Slaw with Apple Cider Mustard Dressing..................111

Simple, Satisfying Meals for Busy Evenings..111
Grilled Chicken Salad with Cauli Rice & Tahini..................112
Eggplant and Mushroom Stir-Fry with Brown Rice..................112
Portobello Mushrooms Stuffed with Quinoa..112
Creamy Amaranth Porridge with Toasted Almonds and Fresh Herbs..................113
Cauliflower Steaks with Garlic and Herb Quinoa..................113
Buckwheat Porridge with Roasted Vegetables and Feta..................113
Ratatouille..................114
Pilaf with Brown Rice..................114
Zucchini Noodles with Pesto and Sautéed Mushrooms..................114
Stuffed Bell Peppers with Ground Turkey and Zucchini..................115
Lentil and Vegetable Skillet with Fresh Herbs..................115
Tofu and Cabbage Stir-Fry with Ginger-Garlic Sauce..................115
Egg and Cauliflower Skillet with Baby Spinach..................116
Stuffed Zucchini Boats with Mushrooms and Feta..................116
Tempeh Stir-Fry with Snow Peas and Ginger..................116
Baked Tofu with Steamed Broccoli and Tahini Sauce..................117
Stuffed Bell Peppers with Ground Turkey and Quinoa..................117
Cabbage Stir-Fry with Eggs and Carrots.117

Fish and Seafood..................118
Grilled Shrimp and Asparagus Salad with Garlic-Lemon Dressing..................118
Baked Salmon with Broccoli and Lemon Dill Sauce..................118
Tuna Niçoise Salad with Hard-Boiled Eggs and Olive Oil..................118
Baked Cod with Roasted Brussels Sprouts..119
Seared Tuna Steak with Avocado and Cucumber Salad..................119
Herb-Crusted Halibut with Cauliflower Mash 119
Broiled Mackerel with Sautéed Spinach..120
Baked Flounder with Broccoli and Cauliflower..................120
Grilled Calamari with Lemon and Arugula Salad..................120
Grilled Octopus with Arugula and Olive Oil...121
Roasted Salmon Cakes with Yogurt Dill Sauce..................121
Baked Trout with Roasted Fennel and Lemon..................121
Grilled Swordfish Steaks with Zucchini Ribbons..................122
Fish Lettuce Tacos with Avocado Lime Sauce..................122
Sardine and Chickpea Salad with Lemon Mustard Dressing..................122
Steamed Cod with Ginger-Garlic Cabbage...123
Grilled Tilapia with Roasted Eggplant and Tomato..................123

Lemon-Parsley Scallops with Sautéed Zucchini 123

Vegetarian and Plant-Based Options to Keep Blood Sugar Steady 124

Roasted Veggie Salad with Pumpkin Seeds & Lemon Vinaigrette 124

Zoodle and Arugula Salad with Lemon-Parmesan Dressing 124

Spinach and Quinoa Salad with Sunflower Seeds and Lemon Zest 124

Avocado and Baby Kale Salad with Cucumber and Herb Dressing 125

Roasted Eggplant Salad with Tahini and Pomegranate 125

Eggplant Rollatini with Ricotta and Spinach.. 125

Cauliflower Tabbouleh with Cucumber, Tomato, and Mint 126

Kale and Quinoa Stuffed Acorn Squash with Tahini Drizzle 126

Lentil and Vegetable Stew with Fresh Herbs 126

Orange and Spinach Salad with Almonds..... 127

Stuffed Bell Peppers with Quinoa, Chickpeas, and Herbs 127

Chickpea and Kale Stir-Fry with Garlic and Lemon 127

Sweet Potato and Black Bean Salad with Lime-Cilantro Dressing 128

Grilled Tofu with Sesame-Ginger Dressing and Broccoli 128

Spaghetti Squash Bowl with Roasted Chickpeas and Spinach 128

Lentil and Sweet Potato Patties with Herb Yogurt Sauce 129

Stuffed Bell Peppers with Black Beans and Cauliflower Rice 129

Roasted Carrot and Lentil Salad with Lemon-Cumin Dressing 129

Festive Dishes for Special Occasions 130

Seafood Paella with Brown Rice 130

Herb-Roasted Whole Chicken with Garlic and Lemon 130

Roast Duck with Apples and Cinnamon .. 130

Roast Turkey with Herb-Cauliflower Stuffing and Roasted Vegetables 131

Beef Wellington with Almond Flour Crust and Roasted Asparagus 131

Stuffed Turkey Roulade with Cranberry and Almond Filling 131

Spinach & Feta Stuffed Chicken 132

Stuffed Pork Tenderloin with Spinach, Walnuts, and Goat Cheese 132

Shepherd's Pie with Cauliflower Mash 132

Stuffed Bell Peppers with Ground Turkey and Quinoa 133

Walnut-Crusted Chicken with Garlic Green Beans 133

Cauliflower Gratin with Almond Milk and Gruyère 133

Beef and Mushroom Skillet with Rosemary.. 134

Stuffed Acorn Squash with Wild Rice and Cranberries 134

Salmon Fillet with Pomegranate Glaze and Herbs 134

Zucchini Rollatini with Ricotta and Walnut Filling 135

Stuffed Bell Peppers with Lentils and Herbs. 135

Grilled Eggplant Steaks with Herbed Yogurt Sauce 135

CHAPTER 7: BONUSES AND USEFUL MATERIALS 136

60-Day Grocery Shopping Templates for Diabetes 136

Personalized Health Journal 153

Tips for Successful Journaling 154

APPENDIX MEASUREMENT CONVERSION CHART 159

Meet the Author – Andrew Moore 160

EDITOR'S LETTER

Dear Reader,

If you're beginning your path with prediabetes or Type 2, welcome — this book was made for you.

A diagnosis can feel like a lot to take in. But here's the truth: you don't have to give up delicious food, comfort, or joy. With the right support and practical tools, you can take back control—starting now.

Why This Cookbook Stands Out

*✓ **365+ Days of Blood Sugar-Friendly Recipes** — easy, balanced meals you can make in 30 minutes or less, all designed to help stabilize glucose naturally.*

*✓ **No Trendy Tricks** — just simple, nourishing food to support your energy, mood, and long-term health.*

*✓ **Low-Carb, Low-Sugar, High Flavor** — crafted to manage blood sugar effectively while keeping every bite satisfying.*

*✓ **Everyday Ingredients, Real-Life Cooking** — no complicated products or confusing methods. Just what you need, with clear directions.*

*✓ **60-Day Meal Plan to Jumpstart Your Routine** — no more confusion, just a realistic, supportive guide to better habits and feeling your best.*

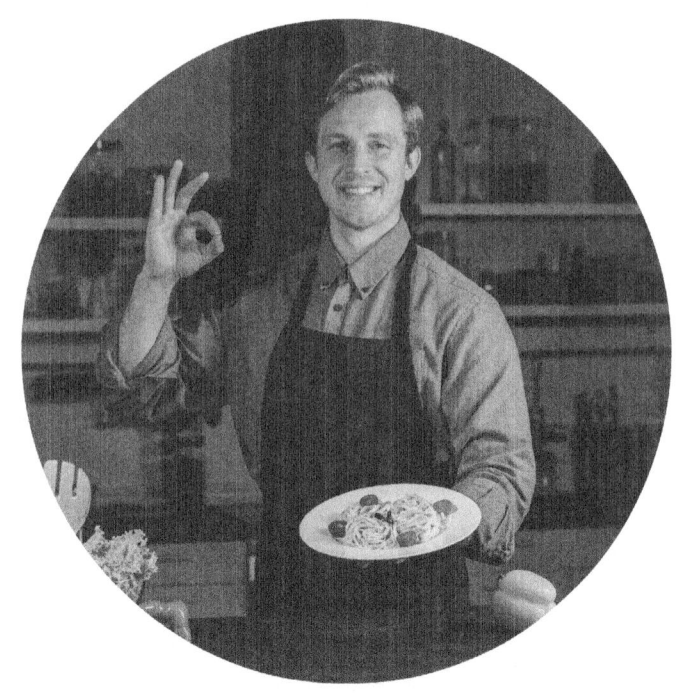

Whether you've been recently diagnosed, supporting a loved one, or simply want to eat healthier, this book is here to empower and encourage you.

Healthy eating doesn't have to feel like a burden. It can be enjoyable, comforting, and deeply rewarding. I hope this book becomes a trusted part of your kitchen—and your wellness journey—for years to come.

With gratitude,
Andrew Moore

Follow Andrew Moore on Amazon for new releases, exclusive recipes, and helpful tips!

CHAPTER 1: GETTING STARTED — THE ESSENTIALS OF DIABETES & HEALTHY EATING

Welcome to Chapter One, where we'll break down the core facts about diabetes and nutrition, offering clear insights to help you make smart choices for your well-being.

Understanding the Types of Diabetes

Type 1 diabetes often develops early in life and happens when the pancreas can't make enough insulin. Without insulin, the body can't use sugar for energy. People with Type 1 need insulin from outside sources to keep their blood sugar stable.

Type 2 diabetes is more commonly linked to lifestyle—things like diet, weight, and activity levels. The pancreas may still produce insulin, but the body doesn't respond to it well. This form of diabetes is often manageable with nutrition, movement, and daily habits.

Prediabetes means blood sugar levels are higher than normal but not yet in the Type 2 range. It's a critical early warning sign and an opportunity to take action before diabetes fully develops.

Why Diabetes Happens: Getting to the Root

Knowing the reasons behind a diabetes diagnosis is key to making lasting lifestyle changes.

Genes and Lifestyle Working Together:

While Type 2 diabetes can run in families, genes aren't the full picture. Some people are more likely to get it based on genetics—but how we live has a major impact. Food choices, stress, and movement all play important roles in diabetes risk.

How Extra Weight & Inactivity Contribute:

One of the biggest drivers of Type 2 is excess fat, especially around the stomach. This can lead to insulin resistance—when cells stop reacting to insulin and sugar stays in the blood.

Sitting too much and not moving enough also raise the risk. Without physical activity, it's harder to burn sugar or fat. Exercise helps improve insulin response and supports a healthy weight—both key in preventing or managing diabetes.

Why Regular Movement Matters for Diabetes

Staying active is one of the easiest and most effective ways to lower your risk of Type 2 diabetes. Regular movement offers a wide range of health benefits. First, it helps manage weight by burning calories and building lean muscle — both key in keeping blood sugar steady. A healthy weight makes it easier for your body to use insulin the way it should.

Exercise also boosts insulin sensitivity. When you do things like walking, dancing, or swimming, your cells respond better to insulin. That means your body can move sugar out of the blood more efficiently — a big win for anyone dealing with insulin resistance.

Finally, physical activity protects your heart. Since diabetes raises the risk of heart issues, staying active strengthens your cardiovascular system, improves circulation, and helps prevent future complications.

The Role of a Balanced Plate in Preventing Diabetes

Eating well is just as powerful as staying active. A diet full of whole grains, vegetables, fruits, lean protein, and healthy fats gives your body what it needs—without spiking your blood sugar. These foods are packed with nutrients and help keep your energy stable throughout the day.

Fiber is especially helpful. It improves digestion, helps with weight control, and slows sugar absorption. That's why fiber-rich meals are key for managing blood sugar levels.

Try to avoid sugary drinks, overly processed snacks, and refined carbs. These foods make your blood sugar jump, put stress on your body, and can lead to long-term complications if eaten too often.

Eating Made Simple: What to Choose for Better Blood Sugar

Low-GI Foods: A Simple Foundation

The Glycemic Index (GI) helps you choose carbs that won't spike your blood sugar. Low-GI foods break down slowly, so sugar enters your bloodstream more gradually. That's what makes them perfect for a diabetes-friendly lifestyle.

Look for foods like quinoa, barley, and oats. Pair them with non-starchy veggies like broccoli, spinach, and cauliflower. Legumes like lentils and chickpeas are another smart choice—they're rich in both fiber and protein.

Skip the Sugar Crash: Avoid These Traps

High-sugar and high-carb foods can lead to a blood sugar rollercoaster—first a spike, then a crash. This can make managing diabetes harder and leave you feeling drained.

Avoid soda, packaged sweets, and refined carbs like white bread or sugary cereals. Instead, pick natural options like monk fruit or allulose when you want something sweet.

Also, cut back on things like white flour, baked goods, and sweet breakfast foods. These break down fast and cause sudden glucose spikes—exactly what you want to avoid.

Must-Know Nutrition Tips: Reading Labels That Matter

Spotting Hidden Sugars and Carbs

Learning to read food labels is essential for keeping carbs and sugars under control. Ingredients like sugar often go by other names—making it harder to spot them.

Watch for words like "sucrose," "fructose," and "corn syrup." These are added sugars that can sneak into your diet if you're not careful.

Ingredients to Limit or Avoid for Better Blood Sugar

Sugars and Their Hidden Forms:

- Sucrose
- Fructose
- Glucose
- Corn Syrup
- Honey
- Maltodextrin

Fast-Digesting Carbs and Refined Grains:

- White flour
- Potato starch
- Rice
- Bread
- Dough
- Potatoes

Unhealthy Fats:

- Hydrogenated oils
- Trans fats
- Palm oil

Too Much Salt:

Eating a lot of sodium can raise blood pressure and increase the risk of heart disease. Keep salty foods in check.

Watch Out for Sneaky Additives:

Flavorings and additives (even the "natural" ones) can hide extra sugars or carbs. Always check the label.

Preservatives:

Some preservatives can disrupt blood sugar control — especially when found in packaged snacks.

Artificial Sweeteners to Be Cautious With:

- Aspartame
- Sucralose
- Saccharin
- Acesulfame Potassium

This list is a general guideline — always consult your doctor for personalized advice. Read ingredient lists carefully and stay mindful of sugar, carbs, and unhealthy fats in everyday products.

Choosing the Right Foods for Energy & Health

Focus on foods that nourish your body without spiking your blood sugar. Bright-colored vegetables like spinach, peppers, and carrots are packed with nutrients and naturally low in carbs.

Add lean proteins such as chicken, tofu, beans, and eggs. They help you stay full, support muscle repair, and slow down sugar absorption when eaten with carbs — a win-win for blood sugar balance.

Smart Ingredient Picks for Diabetic-Friendly Meals

Lean & Healthy Proteins:

- Chicken
- Turkey
- Fish
- Eggs
- Tofu
- Almond Butter

Low-Fat Dairy:

- Skim Milk
- Low-Fat Yogurt
- Low-Fat Cottage Cheese

Low-Carb Carbs (Yes, Really!):

- Quinoa
- Brown Rice
- Non-starchy Vegetables
- Low-sugar Fruits (like berries or citrus)

Good Fats That Work for You:

- Olive Oil
- Avocado
- Nuts

Better Sweet Choices:

- Allulose
- Monk Fruit
- Honey (in small amounts)

Fiber for the Win:
Dietary fiber helps slow sugar absorption, supports digestion, and keeps you feeling full longer.

Low-Sugar Pantry Staples:

- Raw nuts and seeds
- Unsweetened dairy (like plain yogurt)
- 100% natural juices (no added sugar)

This list is your go-to for building blood sugar–friendly meals. Always adjust based on your needs and talk to a doctor or dietitian when needed.

Simple Kitchen Tips to Keep Blood Sugar Balanced

Choosing the right ingredients is only part of the story. How you cook makes a big difference, too! Try these easy, diabetes-friendly methods:

How to Cook Without Spiking Sugar

Steam, Don't Boil:
Steaming preserves nutrients and flavor better than boiling, which can wash away important vitamins.

Roast & Grill:
Roasting brings out natural sweetness in veggies, while grilling adds bold flavor without added fat.

Quick Sauté:
Stir-frying with a small amount of olive oil over high heat helps seal in texture and nutrients fast.

Slow & Steady:
Slow cooking is great for stews and soups—it keeps flavors rich and nutrients intact.

Microwave Smart:
Microwaving can actually be nutrient-friendly if

done right. Use minimal water and microwave-safe containers.

Easy Ingredient Swaps That Make a Big Difference

Whole Grains Over Refined Ones:
Pick brown rice, quinoa, or whole wheat pasta instead of white versions—they're lower GI and richer in fiber.

Heart-Healthy Fats:
Ditch saturated fats (like butter) and go for olive oil, avocado, or nuts to support heart and blood sugar health.

Use Better Sweeteners:
Go with natural sweeteners like monk fruit or allulose to enjoy sweetness without the sugar spike.

Make Meals Work Harder for You

Choose Lean Proteins:
Poultry, tofu, legumes, and fish give you nutrients without extra cholesterol. Great with any meal!

Stick With Low-Fat Dairy:
Choose options like low-fat yogurt or cottage cheese to get calcium and vitamin D without added fats.

Portion Smart:
Even healthy foods can spike blood sugar if the portions are too big. Use smaller plates to stay in control.

Small cooking changes and smart swaps can transform your kitchen into a diabetes-friendly zone. It's not just about cutting sugar—it's about making meals that truly support your health and make you feel great every day.

CHAPTER 2: 60-DAY MEAL PLAN

Day	Breakfast	Lunch	Snack	Dinner
Day 1	Turkey Sausage and Veggie Scramble – p.21	Beef and Vegetable Stew with Carrots and Celery – p.49	Cucumber Slices with Avocado and Hummus – p.78	Kale and Spinach Salad with Balsamic Vinaigrette and Feta – p.106
Day 2	Almond Butter Couscous Porridge with Blueberries and Flaxseeds – p.31	Quinoa Bowl with Grilled Chicken and Roasted Peppers – p.57	Keto Pumpkin Pie Bites with Coconut Cream – p.92	Stuffed Bell Peppers with Ground Turkey and Zucchini – p.115
Day 3	Egg-Stuffed Bell Pepper Boats – p.47	Creamy Mushroom Soup with Roasted Garlic and Herbs – p.52	Celery Sticks with Almond Butter and Chia Seeds – p.82	Grilled Tilapia with Roasted Eggplant and Tomato – p.123
Day 4	Cauliflower Rice Stir-Fry with Scrambled Eggs and Garlic – p.43	Spelt Bowl with Sautéed Kale and Poached Egg – p.62	Sugar-Free Raspberry Mousse with Whipped Coconut Cream – p.94	Grilled Shrimp and Asparagus Salad with Garlic-Lemon Dressing – p.118
Day 5	Low-Carb Cottage Cheese and Spinach Pancakes – p.38	Garlic Turkey Meatball Soup with Greens – p.55	Cottage Cheese with Sliced Tomatoes and Cucumber – p.85	Zoodle and Arugula Salad with Lemon-Parmesan Dressing – p.124
Day 6	Coconut Yogurt Parfait with Berries and Seeds – p.46	Barley Bowl with Grilled Tofu and Red Cabbage – p.61	Cinnamon Vanilla Chia Custard – p.97	Cauliflower Tabbouleh with Mint and Lemon Vinaigrette – p.107
Day 7	Kale and Coconut Protein Bowl – p.31	Barley and Mushroom Bowl with Baby Kale – p.57	Turkey and Cheese Skewers with Olives – p.85	Grilled Swordfish Steaks with Zucchini Ribbons – p.122
Day 8	Berry Almond Quinoa Bowl – p.27	Tomato and Red Lentil Soup with Fresh Basil – p.53	Hard-Boiled Eggs with Olive Tapenade – p.83	Chicken Thighs with Dijon-Caper Sauce – p.76
Day 9	Egg White and Turkey Sausage Scramble – p.35	Chicken and Cauliflower Rice Casserole with Broccoli – p.64	Low-Sugar Apple Spice Cake with Almond Flour – p.99	Salmon Fillet with Pomegranate Glaze and Herbs – p.134
Day 10	Crustless Veggie Quiche with Bell Peppers and Onions – p.42	Vegetable and Ground Beef Stew with Zucchini – p.51	Almond Flour Snickerdoodle Cookies – p.94	Grilled Eggplant Salad with Yogurt-Tahini Dressing – p.111
Day 11	Avocado and Chia Seed Smoothie – p.32	Freekeh Bowl with Roasted Brussels Sprouts and Tahini Drizzle – p.60	Mini Chocolate Hazelnut Cakes – p.104	Beef Wellington with Almond Flour Crust and Roasted Asparagus – p.131
Day 12	Buckwheat Pancakes with Cinnamon and Walnuts – p.45	Turkey and Spinach Soup with Lemon – p.54	Blueberry Almond Mug Cake – p.95	Herb-Crusted Halibut with Cauliflower Mash – p.119

Day	Breakfast	Lunch	Snack	Dinner
Day 13	Mushroom and Asparagus Egg Bake – p.42	Eggplant Moussaka with Ground Beef and Parmesan – p.63	Keto Lemon Bars with Coconut Crust – p.92	Roasted Eggplant Salad with Tahini and Pomegranate – p.125
Day 14	Pumpkin and Cinnamon Smoothie – p.29	Creamy Cauliflower and Leek Soup with Roasted Garlic – p.49	Orange Almond Biscotti – p.103	Grilled Chicken Salad with Cauli Rice & Tahini – p.112
Day 15	Cottage Cheese Omelet with Herbs – p.41	Eggplant Chickpea Stew with Tahini – p.55	Cottage Cheese with Walnuts and Cinnamon – p.84	Grilled Octopus with Arugula and Olive Oil – p.121
Day 16	Grilled Steak with Roasted Vegetables and Quinoa – p.37	Creamy Broccoli and Cauliflower Soup with Almonds – p.49	Keto Chocolate Lava Cake with Dark Chocolate Filling – p.93	Spinach & Feta Stuffed Chicken – p.132
Day 17	Tofu Scramble with Peppers and Spinach – p.27	Buckwheat and Roasted Broccoli Bowl with Sunflower Seeds – p.57	Avocado & Egg Mash on Zucchini Rounds – p.89	Lentil and Vegetable Skillet with Fresh Herbs – p.115
Day 18	Keto Pumpkin Pancakes with Pecans – p.44	Chicken and Lentil Stew – p.50	Coconut Matcha Energy Balls – p.94	Seared Duck Breast with Red Cabbage and Caraway – p.77
Day 19	Spinach and Mushroom Egg Muffins – p.25	Buckwheat Bowl with Smoked Salmon and Avocado – p.61	Ricotta-Stuffed Sweet Mini Peppers – p.88	Stuffed Pork Tenderloin with Spinach, Walnuts, and Goat Cheese – p.132
Day 20	Almond Flour Crepes with Ricotta and Spinach – p.44	Quinoa and Roasted Veggie Bowl with Tahini Dressing – p.58	Mini Lemon Ricotta Cups with Coconut Crust – p.96	Baked Flounder with Broccoli and Cauliflower – p.120
Day 21	Zucchini and Feta Omelet – p.26	Green Vegetable Stew with Chicken and Dill – p.53	Tuna-Stuffed Avocados with Olive Oil and Lemon – p.86	Cauliflower Steaks with Garlic and Herb Quinoa – p.113
Day 22	Strawberry Almond Breakfast Smoothie – p.33	Quinoa and Black Bean Bowl with Cilantro-Lime Yogurt – p.62	Keto-Friendly Berry Cheesecake Bars – p.91	Grilled Calamari with Lemon and Arugula Salad – p.120
Day 23	Spinach and Feta Scramble with a Side of Sautéed Mushrooms – p.23	Chicken and Quinoa Soup with Spinach and Herbs – p.50	Almond Coconut Ice Cream Bites – p.103	Broccoli and Chickpea Salad with Garlic Yogurt Dressing – p.109
Day 24	Pumpkin Spice Quinoa Porridge with Almond Milk – p.30	Buckwheat Bowl with Grilled Chicken and Avocado – p.58	Chicken Salad with Avocado and Chia Seeds – p.87	Baked Tofu with Steamed Broccoli and Tahini Sauce – p.117
Day 25	Savory Quinoa Breakfast Bowl – p.25	Beef and Barley Soup with Root Vegetables – p.51	Banana Nut Oat Bars with Almond Butter – p.95	Roasted Beet and Goat Cheese Salad with Balsamic Glaze – p.108

Day	Breakfast	Lunch	Snack	Dinner
Day 26	Sautéed Zucchini and Bell Pepper Frittata – p.23	Farro and Grilled Vegetables with a Yogurt-Tahini Dressing – p.56	Spinach Egg Bites with Cottage Cheese – p.87	Sweet Potato and Black Bean Salad with Lime-Cilantro Dressing – p.128
Day 27	Spinach and Feta Stuffed Chicken Breasts – p.34	Eggplant & Chicken Casserole with Herb Yogurt – p.67	Pumpkin Hummus with Cucumber – p.80	Roasted Cauliflower and Chickpea Salad with Tahini-Garlic Dressing – p.110
Day 28	Chia Seed Pudding with Coconut Milk and Raspberries – p.22	Barley and Roasted Red Pepper Bowl with Turkey – p.59	Turkey and Avocado Lettuce Wraps – p.86	Cabbage Stir-Fry with Eggs and Carrots – p.117
Day 29	Blueberry Spinach Smoothie with Flaxseeds – p.31	Spinach and Feta Crustless Quiche with Almond Flour – p.63	Egg and Veggie Cups with Bell Pepper and Onion – p.89	Ratatouille – p.114
Day 30	Cottage Cheese with Fresh Peaches and a Drizzle of Honey – p.21	Chard and Ricotta Bake with Tomato Slices – p.68	Cacao Coconut Bites with Allulose – p.95	Spinach and Strawberry Salad with Poppy Seed Dressing – p.108
Day 31	High-Protein Dishes to Stabilize Blood Sugar – p.34	Farro Bowl with Roasted Butternut Squash and Chicken – p.59	Stuffed Cherry Tomatoes with Avocado and Tuna – p.84	Grilled Tofu with Sesame-Ginger Dressing and Broccoli – p.128
Day 32	Avocado and Tofu Breakfast Bowl – p.26	Butternut Squash and Zucchini Lasagna with Turkey and Ricotta – p.65	Chicken & Avocado Pita Wedges – p.88	Avocado and Cucumber Salad with Lime-Cilantro Dressing – p.110
Day 33	Grilled Chicken Salad with Avocado and Quinoa – p.35	Grilled Turkey Tenderloin with Roasted Vegetables – p.70	Tofu Salad with Greens and Lemon-Oil Dressing – p.89	Steamed Cod with Ginger-Garlic Cabbage – p.123
Day 34	Cucumber and Kale Smoothie – p.28	Zucchini and Herb Soup with Poached Egg – p.55	Zucchini Chips with Parmesan Dust – p.82	Spaghetti Squash Bowl with Roasted Chickpeas and Spinach – p.128
Day 35	Hard-Boiled Eggs with Avocado and Spinach Salad – p.21	Spaghetti Squash Casserole with Chicken and Alfredo Sauce – p.65	No-Bake Coconut Almond Bars – p.97	Broccoli and Avocado Salad with Lemon-Garlic Dressing – p.111
Day 36	Egg Muffins with Bell Peppers and Spinach – p.24	Tofu and Mushroom Crustless Pie with Herbs – p.68	Lemon Poppy Seed Muffins with Almond Flour – p.93	Cauliflower Gratin with Almond Milk and Gruyère – p.133
Day 37	Mini Broccoli and Cheese Casserole – p.47	Root Vegetable and Beef Stew with Fresh Parsley – p.52	Coconut Chia Pudding with Berries – p.90	Grilled Turkey and Mixed Greens Salad with Mustard Vinaigrette – p.108
Day 38	Warm Kale and Quinoa Breakfast Bowl with Soft-Boiled Egg – p.24	Mushroom and Ground Beef Casserole with Cauliflower – p.65	Kale and Spinach Hummus with Almond Flour Crackers – p.79	Stuffed Bell Peppers with Black Beans and Cauliflower Rice – p.129

Day	Breakfast	Lunch	Snack	Dinner
Day 39	Zucchini and Egg Casserole with Feta and Oregano – p.42	Grilled Flank Steak with Quinoa and Roasted Brussels Sprouts – p.71	Banana Almond Mug Muffin – p.96	Orange and Spinach Salad with Almonds – p.127
Day 40	Savory Greek Bowl with Eggs and Olives – p.32	Zucchini and Mushroom Lasagna with Ricotta and Mozzarella – p.64	Low-Carb Whole Grain Pita with Basil Pesto and Feta – p.81	Baked Chicken Drumsticks with Veggie Sauté – p.77
Day 41	Asparagus and Goat Cheese Omelette with Fresh Herbs – p.23	Turkey Meatloaf Roll with Mushrooms – p.72	Strawberry and Coconut Cream Chia Parfait – p.93	Eggplant Rollatini with Ricotta and Spinach – p.125
Day 42	Zucchini and Egg Protein Bowl – p.32	Chicken and Chickpea Salad with Avocado and Lime – p.36	Radish Slices with Herbed Cream Cheese – p.84	Walnut-Crusted Chicken with Garlic Green Beans – p.133
Day 43	Sweet Potato and Spinach Hash with Egg – p.26	French-Style Baked Meat – p.70	Beetroot Hummus with Carrot and Zucchini Ribbons – p.80	Chickpea and Kale Stir-Fry with Garlic and Lemon – p.127
Day 44	Cauliflower and Egg Power Bowl – p.33	Grilled Sirloin with Cauli Rice & Asparagus – p.72	Stuffed Bell Peppers with Quinoa, Chickpeas, and Herbs – p.127	Grilled Eggplant Steaks with Herbed Yogurt Sauce – p.135
Day 45	Eggplant Breakfast Pizza with Scrambled Eggs and Parmesan – p.45	Cabbage and Tofu Bake with Almond Crumble – p.67	Avocado Tuna Boats – p.82	Baked Trout with Roasted Fennel and Lemon – p.121
Day 46	Apple Cinnamon Overnight Oats with Flaxseeds – p.22	Beef Roll with Spinach, Feta & Eggplant – p.73	Low-Carb Strawberry Shortcake Cups – p.104	Pilaf with Brown Rice – p.114
Day 47	Nutty Green Smoothie with Zucchini and Almonds – p.33	Crustless Zucchini Pie with Goat Cheese and Dill – p.69	Spinach and Ricotta Stuffed Mushrooms – p.79	Cauliflower Tabbouleh with Cucumber, Tomato, and Mint – p.126
Day 48	Eggplant and Goat Cheese Stack – p.48	Pork Loin with Apple & Sage – p.73	Olive and Sun-Dried Tomato Hummus with Zucchini – p.80	Roasted Salmon Cakes with Yogurt Dill Sauce – p.121
Day 49	Turkey and Cabbage Stir-Fry – p.41	Brussels Sprouts and Chicken Casserole with Almond Crust – p.69	Sliced Chicken Breast with Guacamole and Veggies – p.85	Herb-Roasted Whole Chicken with Garlic and Lemon – p.130
Day 50	Soft-Boiled Eggs with Sautéed Kale and Mushrooms – p.34	Bulgur Wheat Bowl with Ground Turkey and Zucchini – p.56	Turkey and Cucumber Roll-Ups with Mustard Dip – p.88	Lemon-Parsley Scallops with Sautéed Zucchini – p.123
Day 51	Chicken and Chickpea Salad with Avocado and Lime – p.36	Butternut Squash and Turkey Chili – p.50	Deviled Eggs with Smoked Salmon and Avocado Mousse – p.81	Broiled Mackerel with Sautéed Spinach – p.120

Day	Breakfast	Lunch	Snack	Dinner
Day 52	Turkey and Black Bean Chili with Avocado – p.37	Millet and Carrot Bowl with Turkey Meatballs – p.56	Smoked Salmon Rolls with Cucumber and Cream Cheese – p.83	Stuffed Acorn Squash with Wild Rice and Cranberries – p.134
Day 53	Baked Zucchini Turkey Fritters – p.46	Millet and Roasted Cauliflower Bowl with Lemon Vinaigrette – p.58	Coconut Flour Vanilla Cupcakes with Greek Yogurt Frosting – p.105	Tuna Niçoise Salad with Hard-Boiled Eggs and Olive Oil – p.118
Day 54	Turkey and Veggie Breakfast Patties – p.27	Cabbage and Beef Tomato Stew – p.54	Strawberry Coconut Yogurt Bark – p.96	Shepherd's Pie with Cauliflower Mash – p.132
Day 55	Low-Carb Zucchini Fritters with Poached Eggs – p.44	Spinach and Quinoa Salad with Sunflower Seeds and Lemon Zest – p.124	Coconut Flour Banana Bread with Chia Seeds – p.100	Egg and Cauliflower Skillet with Baby Spinach – p.116
Day 56	Warm Chia Almond Porridge with Berries – p.47	Ground Turkey and Kale Casserole with Almond Crust – p.64	Cilantro Lime Hummus with Bell Pepper Strips – p.81	Broccoli and Turkey Breakfast Bake with Cheddar – p.67
Day 57	Egg and Spinach Breakfast Muffins with Turkey Bacon – p.36	Creamy Turnip and Leek Soup – p.54	Keto-Friendly Lemon Coconut Cake – p.100	Tofu and Cabbage Stir-Fry with Ginger-Garlic Sauce – p.115
Day 58	Buckwheat Porridge with Almonds and Raspberries – p.30	Barley Bowl with Roasted Fennel and Chicken – p.62	Sugar-Free Pumpkin Spice Cupcakes with Cream Cheese Frosting – p.99	Crustless Zucchini Pie with Goat Cheese and Dill – p.69
Day 59	Crustless Quiche with Spinach, Mushrooms, and Feta – p.46	Savory Beef and Mushroom Stew with Fresh Thyme – p.52	Keto Maple Pecan Scones – p.102	Zucchini Rollatini with Ricotta and Walnut Filling – p.135
Day 60	Broccoli and Cheddar Scramble with Herbs – p.34	Amaranth and Mushroom Bowl with Herb Yogurt Sauce – p.60	Coconut Raspberry Thumbprint Cookies – p.104	Grilled Sirloin with Cauli Rice & Asparagus – p.72

Note: We wish to remind you that the 60-Day Meal Plan provided in this book is intended as a guide and a source of inspiration. The caloric content of the dishes is approximate and may vary depending on the portion sizes and specific ingredients. This plan represents a diverse, balanced menu, combining a richness of proteins, healthy fats, and minimal carbohydrates. It allows for following a low-carb diet while enjoying delicious and nutritious meals every day.

If you find that the calories in the recipes do not completely align with your personal needs or the plan, feel free to adjust the portion sizes. Increase or decrease them to ensure that the meal plan suits your individual goals and preferences. Be creative and enjoy each dish according to your needs!

CHAPTER 3: BREAKFAST: Quick and Easy Diabetic-Friendly Breakfast Ideas

Turkey Sausage and Veggie Scramble

Prep: 10 minutes | **Cook:** 10 minutes | **Serves:** 2

Ingredients:

- 4 oz turkey sausage, crumbled (115g)
- 4 large eggs (200g)
- 1 tbsp olive oil (15g)
- 1/2 cup diced bell peppers (75g)
- 1/2 cup chopped spinach (75g)
- 1/4 tsp ground black pepper (1g)
- 1/8 tsp salt (0.5g)

Instructions:

1. Heat olive oil in a pan over medium heat. Add turkey sausage and cook until browned, about 5 minutes.
2. Add diced bell peppers and cook for 3 minutes until softened.
3. Add chopped spinach and cook for another minute until wilted.
4. Whisk eggs with black pepper and salt. Pour the eggs into the pan and scramble with the vegetables and sausage until fully cooked. Serve warm.

Nutritional Facts (Per Serving): Calories: 400 | Carbohydrates: 6g | Protein: 21g | Fat: 17g | Sugars: 2g | Fiber: 2g | Sodium: 480mg

Glycemic Index: Turkey sausage: Low (GI = 28) | Bell peppers: Low (GI = 15) | Eggs: Negligible GI | Spinach: Low (GI = 15)

Hard-Boiled Eggs with Avocado and Spinach Salad

Prep: 10 minutes | **Cook:** 10 minutes | **Serves:** 2

Ingredients:

- 4 large eggs (200g)
- 1 small avocado (120g)
- 2 cups baby spinach (60g)
- 1 tbsp lemon juice (15ml)
- 1 tbsp olive oil (15ml)
- 1/4 tsp salt (1g)
- 1/8 tsp black pepper (0.5g)

Instructions:

1. Hard-boil the eggs by placing them in boiling water for 9-10 minutes. Let them cool, then peel and halve.
2. In a bowl, toss baby spinach with lemon juice, olive oil, salt, and black pepper.
3. Slice the avocado and arrange it on top of the spinach.
4. Add the hard-boiled egg halves and serve.

Nutritional Facts (Per Serving): Calories: 400 | Carbohydrates: 7g | Protein: 20g | Fat: 17g | Sugars: 2g | Fiber: 6g | Sodium: 340mg

Glycemic Index: Eggs: Negligible GI | Avocado: Low (GI = 15) | Spinach: Low (GI = 15) | Lemon juice: Negligible GI

Cottage Cheese with Fresh Peaches and a Drizzle of Honey

Prep: 5 minutes | **Cook:** None | **Serves:** 2

Ingredients:

- 1 cup low-fat cottage cheese (225g)
- 1 medium peach, sliced (150g)
- 1 tsp honey (5ml)
- 1 tbsp chopped almonds (15g)

Instructions:

1. Divide cottage cheese evenly between two bowls.
2. Top with peach slices and drizzle with honey.
3. Sprinkle with chopped almonds and serve.

Nutritional Facts (Per Serving): Calories: 400 | Carbohydrates: 23g | Protein: 21g | Fat: 13g | Sugars: 5g | Fiber: 3g | Sodium: 320mg

Glycemic Index: Cottage cheese: Low (GI = 27) | Peach: Medium (GI = 42) | Honey: Medium (GI = 58)

Apple Cinnamon Overnight Oats with Flaxseeds

Prep: 5 minutes | **Cook:** None (overnight) | **Serves:** 2

Ingredients:

- 1/2 cup rolled oats (45g)
- 3/4 cup unsweetened almond milk (180ml)
- 1/4 cup plain Greek yogurt (60g)
- 1 tbsp ground flaxseeds (10g)
- 1/2 tsp cinnamon (1g)
- 1/2 medium apple, diced (75g)
- 1 tsp low carb sweetener (5g)

Instructions:

1. In a jar or bowl, combine oats, almond milk, Greek yogurt, flaxseeds, cinnamon, and low carb sweetener. Stir well.
2. Add diced apple on top. Cover and refrigerate overnight.
3. In the morning, stir the mixture and serve chilled.

Nutritional Facts (Per Serving): Calories: 400 | Carbohydrates: 28g | Protein: 19g | Fat: 14g | Sugars: 5g | Fiber: 7g | Sodium: 310mg

Glycemic Index: Oats: Medium (GI = 55) | Apple: Medium (GI = 38) | Almond milk: Low (GI = 30)

Chia Seed Pudding with Coconut Milk and Raspberries

Prep: 5 minutes | **Cook:** None (overnight) | **Serves:** 2

Ingredients:

- 1/4 cup chia seeds (40g)
- 1 cup unsweetened coconut milk (240ml)
- 1/4 cup plain Greek yogurt (60g)
- 1/2 cup fresh raspberries (60g)
- 1 tsp low carb sweetener (5g)
- 1/2 tsp vanilla extract (2.5ml)

Instructions:

1. In a bowl, whisk together chia seeds, coconut milk, Greek yogurt, low carb sweetener, and vanilla extract.
2. Refrigerate overnight until it thickens.
3. In the morning, top with fresh raspberries and serve.

Nutritional Facts (Per Serving): Calories: 400 | Carbohydrates: 16g | Protein: 18g | Fat: 17g | Sugars: 4g | Fiber: 10g | Sodium: 320mg

Glycemic Index: Chia seeds: Low (GI = 1) | Raspberries: Low (GI = 32) | Coconut milk: Low (GI = 40)

Greek Yogurt Parfait with Walnuts and Mixed Berries

Prep: 5 minutes | **Cook:** None | **Serves:** 2

Ingredients:

- 1 cup plain Greek yogurt (240g)
- 1/4 cup walnuts, chopped (30g)
- 1/2 cup mixed berries (blueberries, strawberries, raspberries) (75g)
- 1 tsp low carb sweetener (5g)
- 1 tbsp flaxseeds (10g)

Instructions:

1. In two bowls, layer Greek yogurt and mixed berries.
2. Top with chopped walnuts, flaxseeds, and low carb sweetener. Serve chilled.

Nutritional Facts (Per Serving): Calories: 400 | Carbohydrates: 21g | Protein: 20g | Fat: 15g | Sugars: 5g | Fiber: 6g | Sodium: 330mg

Glycemic Index: Greek yogurt: Low (GI = 35) | Mixed berries: Low (GI = 40) | Walnuts: Low (GI = 15)

Spinach and Feta Scramble with a Side of Sautéed Mushrooms

Prep: 5 minutes | Cook: 10 minutes | Serves: 2

Ingredients:

- 4 large eggs (200g)
- 1 cup baby spinach (30g)
- 1/4 cup crumbled feta cheese (60g)
- 1 tbsp olive oil (15ml)
- 1 cup sliced mushrooms (100g)
- 1/4 tsp black pepper (1g)
- 1/8 tsp salt (0.5g)

Instructions:

1. In a pan, heat 1/2 tbsp olive oil over medium heat and sauté mushrooms for 5 minutes until golden. Set aside.
2. In the same pan, heat remaining olive oil. Add baby spinach and cook for 1 minute until wilted.
3. Whisk eggs with black pepper and salt, pour into the pan, and scramble with spinach.
4. Add crumbled feta and cook until eggs are fully set.
5. Serve the scramble with the sautéed mushrooms on the side.

Nutritional Facts (Per Serving): Calories: 400 | Carbohydrates: 7g | Protein: 21g | Fat: 17g | Sugars: 2g | Fiber: 2g | Sodium: 420mg

Glycemic Index: Eggs: Negligible GI | Spinach: Low (GI = 15) | Mushrooms: Low (GI = 15) | Feta cheese: Low (GI = 15)

Asparagus and Goat Cheese Omelette with Fresh Herbs

Prep: 5 minutes | Cook: 10 minutes | Serves: 2

Ingredients:

- 4 large eggs (200g)
- 1/2 cup cooked asparagus, chopped (75g)
- 2 tbsp goat cheese, crumbled (30g)
- 1 tbsp olive oil (15ml)
- 1 tbsp chopped fresh herbs (parsley, chives) (5g)
- 1/4 tsp black pepper (1g)
- 1/8 tsp salt (0.5g)

Instructions:

1. Heat olive oil in a non-stick pan over medium heat.
2. Whisk eggs with black pepper, salt, and fresh herbs.
3. Pour the eggs into the pan, then evenly distribute the asparagus and goat cheese on top.
4. Cook for 4-5 minutes until the omelette is set. Fold and serve.

Nutritional Facts (Per Serving): Calories: 400 | Carbohydrates: 5g | Protein: 20g | Fat: 17g | Sugars: 2g | Fiber: 2g | Sodium: 370mg

Glycemic Index: Eggs: Negligible GI | Asparagus: Low (GI = 15) | Goat cheese: Low (GI = 15)

Sautéed Zucchini and Bell Pepper Frittata

Prep: 10 minutes | Cook: 15 minutes | Serves: 2

Ingredients:

- 4 large eggs (200g)
- 1/2 cup diced zucchini (75g)
- 1/2 cup diced bell peppers (75g)
- 1 tbsp olive oil (15ml)
- 1/4 tsp black pepper (1g)
- 1/8 tsp salt (0.5g)

Instructions:

1. Preheat oven to 375°F (190°C).
2. Heat olive oil in an oven-safe skillet over medium heat. Sauté zucchini and bell peppers for 5 minutes until softened.
3. In a bowl, whisk eggs with black pepper and salt. Pour over the vegetables in the skillet.
4. Transfer the skillet to the oven and bake for 10 minutes until the frittata is set. Serve warm.

Nutritional Facts (Per Serving): Calories: 400 | Carbohydrates: 7g | Protein: 20g | Fat: 16g | Sugars: 3g | Fiber: 2g | Sodium: 350mg

Glycemic Index: Zucchini: Low (GI = 15) | Bell peppers: Low (GI = 15) | Eggs: Negligible GI

Egg Muffins with Bell Peppers and Spinach

Prep: 10 minutes | **Cook:** 15 minutes | **Serves:** 2

Ingredients:

- 4 large eggs (200g)
- 1/2 cup diced bell peppers (75g)
- 1 cup baby spinach, chopped (30g)
- 1/4 cup shredded low-fat cheese (30g)
- 1 tbsp olive oil (15ml)
- 1/4 tsp black pepper (1g)
- 1/8 tsp salt (0.5g)

Instructions:

1. Preheat oven to 350°F (175°C).
2. In a bowl, whisk eggs, black pepper, and salt.
3. Stir in bell peppers, spinach, and shredded cheese.
4. Grease a muffin tin with olive oil, pour the egg mixture into the cups, and bake for 15 minutes until set.
5. Serve warm.

Nutritional Facts (Per Serving): Calories: 400 | Carbohydrates: 6g | Protein: 20g | Fat: 17g | Sugars: 2g | Fiber: 2g | Sodium: 370mg

Glycemic Index: Eggs: Negligible GI | Bell peppers: Low (GI = 15) | Spinach: Low (GI = 15)

Almond-Crusted Zucchini Fritters with Poached Eggs

Prep: 10 minutes | **Cook:** 20 minutes | **Serves:** 2

Ingredients:

- 2 medium zucchinis, grated (200g)
- 1/4 cup almond flour (30g)
- 2 large eggs (for poaching) (100g)
- 1 large egg, beaten (50g)
- 2 tbsp olive oil (30ml)
- 1/4 tsp black pepper (1g)
- 1/8 tsp salt (0.5g)

Instructions:

1. Grate zucchini and squeeze out excess moisture. Mix with almond flour, beaten egg, black pepper, and salt.
2. Heat olive oil in a pan over medium heat. Form the mixture into small fritters and cook until golden brown, about 3 minutes per side.
3. In a separate pot, poach eggs by simmering water and cracking eggs gently into it, cooking for 3-4 minutes.
4. Serve the fritters with poached eggs on top.

Nutritional Facts (Per Serving): Calories: 400 | Carbohydrates: 7g | Protein: 19g | Fat: 17g | Sugars: 2g | Fiber: 4g | Sodium: 340mg

Glycemic Index: Zucchini: Low (GI = 15) | Almond flour: Low (GI = 15) | Eggs: Negligible GI

Warm Kale and Quinoa Breakfast Bowl with Soft-Boiled Egg

Prep: 10 minutes | **Cook:** 15 minutes | **Serves:** 2

Ingredients:

- 1/2 cup cooked quinoa (85g)
- 1 cup chopped kale (30g)
- 2 large eggs (100g)
- 1 tbsp olive oil (15ml)
- 1 tbsp lemon juice (15ml)
- 1/4 tsp black pepper (1g)
- 1/8 tsp salt (0.5g)

Instructions:

1. Cook quinoa according to package instructions.
2. In a pan, sauté kale with olive oil, lemon juice, salt, and black pepper for 3-4 minutes.
3. Soft-boil the eggs by simmering in water for 6 minutes, then peel.
4. In bowls, layer quinoa, sautéed kale, and top with the soft-boiled eggs. Serve warm.

Nutritional Facts (Per Serving): Calories: 400 | Carbohydrates: 20g | Protein: 19g | Fat: 17g | Sugars: 1g | Fiber: 4g | Sodium: 350mg

Glycemic Index: Quinoa: Low (GI = 53) | Kale: Low (GI = 15) | Eggs: Negligible

Savory Quinoa Breakfast Bowl

Prep: 10 minutes | Cook: 15 minutes | Serves: 1

Ingredients:

- 1/2 cup cooked quinoa (90g)
- 1 large egg (50g)
- 1/4 avocado, sliced (50g)
- 1/2 cup cherry tomatoes, halved (75g)
- 1 tsp olive oil (5ml)
- 1/4 tsp black pepper (1g)
- 1/8 tsp salt (0.5g)

Instructions:

1. Heat olive oil in a small pan over medium heat. Add cherry tomatoes and cook for 3 minutes.
2. In another pan, cook the egg sunny-side up or poached.
3. Place warm quinoa in a bowl. Top with sautéed tomatoes, avocado slices, and the egg.
4. Sprinkle with salt and black pepper.

Nutritional Facts (Per Serving): Calories: 378 | Carbohydrates: 26g | Protein: 20g | Fat: 16g | Sugar: 3g | Fiber: 7g | Sodium: 320mg

Glycemic Index: Quinoa: 53 | Egg: 0 | Avocado: 15 | Cherry tomatoes: 30

Cottage Cheese and Walnut Toast

Prep: 5 minutes | Cook: 5 minutes | Serves: 1

Ingredients:

- 1 slice whole grain toast (30g)
- 1/2 cup low-fat cottage cheese (100g)
- 1 tbsp chopped walnuts (7g)
- 1/2 tsp ground cinnamon (1.5g)
- 1/2 tsp monk fruit sweetener (1g)
- 1/8 tsp salt (0.5g)

Instructions:

1. Toast the bread to desired crispness.
2. Spread cottage cheese evenly over the toast.
3. Sprinkle with chopped walnuts, cinnamon, monk fruit sweetener, and salt.
4. Serve immediately.

Nutritional Facts (Per Serving): Calories: 392 | Carbohydrates: 28g | Protein: 21g | Fat: 15g | Sugar: 4g | Fiber: 5g | Sodium: 400mg

Glycemic Index: Whole grain bread: 50 | Cottage cheese: 10 | Walnuts: 15

Spinach and Mushroom Egg Muffins

Prep: 10 minutes | Cook: 20 minutes | Serves: 2

Ingredients:

- 2 large eggs (100g)
- 1/2 cup chopped spinach (30g)
- 1/4 cup diced mushrooms (40g)
- 1 tbsp grated parmesan cheese (7g)
- 1/2 tsp olive oil spray (2ml)
- 1/4 tsp black pepper (1g)
- 1/8 tsp salt (0.5g)

Instructions:

1. Preheat oven to 375°F (190°C).
2. In a bowl, whisk eggs with salt, pepper, and parmesan.
3. Stir in spinach and mushrooms.
4. Spray 2 muffin tins with olive oil and pour in the egg mixture.
5. Bake for 18–20 minutes or until set.

Nutritional Facts (Per Serving): Calories: 342 | Carbohydrates: 6g | Protein: 22g | Fat: 17g | Sugar: 2g | Fiber: 2g | Sodium: 450mg

Glycemic Index: Eggs: 0 | Spinach: 15 | Mushrooms: 10 | Parmesan: 0

Zucchini and Feta Omelet

Prep: 7 minutes | **Cook:** 10 minutes | **Serves:** 1

Ingredients:

- 2 large eggs (100g)
- 1/2 cup grated zucchini (60g)
- 2 tbsp crumbled feta cheese (30g)
- 1 tsp olive oil (5ml)
- 1/4 tsp dried oregano (0.5g)
- 1/4 tsp black pepper (1g)
- 1/8 tsp salt (0.5g)

Instructions:

1. In a bowl, whisk eggs with salt, pepper, and oregano.
2. Stir in grated zucchini and feta cheese.
3. Heat olive oil in a non-stick skillet over medium heat.
4. Pour mixture into the skillet and cook for 3–4 minutes per side.
5. Serve warm.

Nutritional Facts (Per Serving): Calories: 370 | Carbohydrates: 4g | Protein: 21g | Fat: 17g | Sugar: 2g | Fiber: 1g | Sodium: 430mg

Glycemic Index: Eggs: 0 | Zucchini: 15 | Feta: 0

Avocado and Tofu Breakfast Bowl

Prep: 10 minutes | **Cook:** 10 minutes | **Serves:** 1

Ingredients:

- 1/2 avocado, cubed (70g)
- 1/2 cup firm tofu, cubed (100g)
- 1/2 cup cooked quinoa (90g)
- 1/2 tbsp olive oil (7ml)
- 1/4 tsp garlic powder (0.5g)
- 1/4 tsp black pepper (1g)
- 1/8 tsp salt (0.5g)

Instructions:

1. Heat olive oil in a skillet over medium heat.
2. Add tofu cubes, garlic powder, salt, and pepper. Sauté for 5–6 minutes.
3. In a bowl, layer cooked quinoa, sautéed tofu, and fresh avocado.
4. Mix gently and serve warm.

Nutritional Facts (Per Serving): Calories: 398 | Carbohydrates: 22g | Protein: 20g | Fat: 18g | Sugar: 1g | Fiber: 6g | Sodium: 420mg

Glycemic Index: Quinoa: 53 | Avocado: 15 | Tofu: 15

Sweet Potato and Spinach Hash with Egg

Prep: 10 minutes | **Cook:** 15 minutes | **Serves:** 1

Ingredients:

- 1/2 cup diced sweet potato (75g)
- 1/2 cup chopped spinach (30g)
- 1 large egg (50g)
- 1/2 tbsp olive oil (7ml)
- 1/4 tsp smoked paprika (0.5g)
- 1/4 tsp black pepper (1g)
- 1/8 tsp salt (0.5g)

Instructions:

1. In a skillet, heat olive oil over medium heat. Add sweet potatoes, salt, pepper, and paprika. Cook 8–10 minutes.
2. Stir in spinach and sauté for 1–2 minutes.
3. In a separate pan, cook the egg to desired doneness.
4. Serve egg on top of the hash.

Nutritional Facts (Per Serving): Calories: 392 | Carbohydrates: 27g | Protein: 19g | Fat: 16g | Sugar: 4g | Fiber: 5g | Sodium: 430mg

Glycemic Index: Sweet potato (boiled/diced): 54 | Spinach: 15 | Egg: 0

Tofu Scramble with Peppers and Spinach

Prep: 8 minutes | Cook: 10 minutes | Serves: 1

Ingredients:

- 1/2 cup firm tofu, crumbled (100g)
- 1/2 cup diced bell peppers (75g)
- 1/2 cup chopped spinach (30g)
- 1/2 tbsp olive oil (7ml)
- 1/4 tsp ground turmeric (0.5g)
- 1/4 tsp black pepper (1g)
- 1/8 tsp salt (0.5g)

Instructions:

1. Heat olive oil in a non-stick skillet over medium heat.
2. Add bell peppers and sauté for 3 minutes.
3. Stir in crumbled tofu, turmeric, salt, and pepper. Cook for 4–5 minutes.
4. Add spinach and cook for 2 more minutes.
5. Serve warm.

Nutritional Facts (Per Serving): Calories: 370 | Carbohydrates: 10g | Protein: 20g | Fat: 17g | Sugar: 3g | Fiber: 3g | Sodium: 420mg

Glycemic Index: Tofu: 15 | Bell pepper: 15 | Spinach: 15

Berry Almond Quinoa Bowl

Prep: 5 minutes | Cook: 15 minutes | Serves: 1

Ingredients:

- 1/2 cup cooked quinoa (90g)
- 1/4 cup fresh blueberries (40g)
- 1 tbsp sliced almonds (8g)
- 1/2 tsp ground cinnamon (1.5g)
- 1/2 tsp monk fruit sweetener (1g)
- 1/4 cup unsweetened almond milk (60ml)

Instructions:

1. Reheat cooked quinoa in a saucepan with almond milk.
2. Stir in cinnamon and monk fruit sweetener.
3. Top with blueberries and sliced almonds.
4. Serve warm.

Nutritional Facts (Per Serving): Calories: 385 | Carbohydrates: 27g | Protein: 18g | Fat: 15g | Sugar: 4g | Fiber: 6g | Sodium: 300mg

Glycemic Index: Quinoa: 53 | Blueberries: 25 | Almonds: 10

Turkey and Veggie Breakfast Patties

Prep: 10 minutes | Cook: 12 minutes | Serves: 2

Ingredients:

- 100g ground turkey breast
- 2 tbsp grated zucchini (30g)
- 2 tbsp chopped red bell pepper (30g)
- 1/2 tbsp olive oil (7ml)
- 1/2 tsp dried thyme (1g)
- 1/4 tsp black pepper (1g)
- 1/8 tsp salt (0.5g)

Instructions:

1. In a bowl, combine turkey, zucchini, bell pepper, thyme, salt, and pepper.
2. Form 2 small patties.
3. Heat olive oil in a non-stick skillet and cook patties over medium heat for 5–6 minutes per side.
4. Serve hot with leafy greens if desired.

Nutritional Facts (Per Serving): Calories: 395 | Carbohydrates: 5g | Protein: 21g | Fat: 17g | Sugar: 2g | Fiber: 1g | Sodium: 440mg

Glycemic Index: Turkey: 0 | Zucchini: 15 | Bell pepper: 15

Low-Carb Breakfast Bowls and Smoothies

Creamy Avocado and Spinach Smoothie Bowl with Chia Seeds

Prep: 5 minutes | **Cook:** None | **Serves:** 2

Ingredients:

- 1 small avocado (120g)
- 1 cup baby spinach (30g)
- 1 cup unsweetened almond milk (240ml)
- 1 tbsp chia seeds (10g)
- 1 tbsp low carb sweetener (5g)
- 1/2 tsp vanilla extract (2.5ml)
- 1/4 cup mixed berries, for topping (40g)

Instructions:

1. In a blender, combine avocado, spinach, almond milk, chia seeds, low carb sweetener, and vanilla extract. Blend until smooth.
2. Pour into bowls and top with mixed berries. Serve immediately.

Nutritional Facts (Per Serving): Calories: 400 | Carbohydrates: 14g | Protein: 19g | Fat: 17g | Sugars: 3g | Fiber: 7g | Sodium: 320mg

Glycemic Index: Avocado: Low (GI = 15) | Spinach: Low (GI = 15) | Chia seeds: Low (GI = 1)

Green Keto Smoothie with Coconut Milk and Almond Butter

Prep: 5 minutes | **Cook:** None | **Serves:** 2

Ingredients:

- 1 cup unsweetened coconut milk (240ml)
- 2 tbsp almond butter (32g)
- 1/2 avocado (60g)
- 1 tbsp chia seeds (10g)
- 1 tbsp low carb sweetener (5g)
- 1 cup kale, chopped (30g)

Instructions:

1. Blend coconut milk, almond butter, avocado, chia seeds, low carb sweetener, and kale until smooth.
2. Pour into glasses and serve immediately.

Nutritional Facts (Per Serving): Calories: 400 | Carbohydrates: 12g | Protein: 19g | Fat: 18g | Sugars: 2g | Fiber: 6g | Sodium: 330mg

Glycemic Index: Coconut milk: Low (GI = 40) | Kale: Low (GI = 15) | Almond butter: Low (GI = 20)

Cucumber and Kale Smoothie

Prep: 5 minutes | **Cook:** None | **Serves:** 2

Ingredients:

- 1 medium cucumber, peeled and chopped (150g)
- 1 cup kale, chopped (30g)
- 1 cup unsweetened almond milk (240ml)
- 1 tbsp chia seeds (10g)
- 1 tbsp low carb sweetener (5g)
- 1/2 tsp lemon juice (2.5ml)

Instructions:

1. In a blender, combine cucumber, kale, almond milk, chia seeds, low carb sweetener, and lemon juice.
2. Blend until smooth.
3. Pour into glasses and serve immediately.

Nutritional Facts (Per Serving): Calories: 400 | Carbohydrates: 10g | Protein: 18g | Fat: 17g | Sugars: 2g | Fiber: 6g | Sodium: 300mg

Glycemic Index: Cucumber: Low (GI = 15) | Kale: Low (GI = 15) | Almond milk: Low (GI = 30)

Pumpkin and Cinnamon Smoothie

Prep: 5 minutes | **Cook:** None | **Serves:** 2

Ingredients:

- 1/2 cup pumpkin purée (120g)
- 1 cup unsweetened almond milk (240ml)
- 1 tbsp chia seeds (10g)
- 1/2 tsp ground cinnamon (1g)
- 1 tbsp low carb sweetener (5g)
- 1/2 tsp vanilla extract (2.5ml)

Instructions:

1. In a blender, combine pumpkin purée, almond milk, chia seeds, cinnamon, low carb sweetener, and vanilla extract. Blend until smooth.
2. Pour into glasses and serve immediately.

Nutritional Facts (Per Serving): Calories: 400 | Carbohydrates: 18g | Protein: 19g | Fat: 15g | Sugars: 3g | Fiber: 7g | Sodium: 320mg

Glycemic Index: Pumpkin: Low (GI = 51) | Chia seeds: Low (GI = 1) | Almond milk: Low (GI = 30)

Cinnamon Quinoa Breakfast Bowl with Almonds and Berries

Prep: 10 minutes | **Cook:** 15 minutes | **Serves:** 2

Ingredients:

- 1/2 cup cooked quinoa (85g)
- 1 cup unsweetened almond milk (240ml)
- 1 tbsp chopped almonds (15g)
- 1 tbsp low carb sweetener (5g)
- 1/2 tsp ground cinnamon (1g)
- 1/2 cup mixed berries (75g)

Instructions:

1. In a small pot, combine cooked quinoa, almond milk, cinnamon, and low carb sweetener. Simmer for 5 minutes until thickened.
2. Serve in bowls, topped with chopped almonds and mixed berries.

Nutritional Facts (Per Serving): Calories: 400 | Carbohydrates: 20g | Protein: 19g | Fat: 16g | Sugars: 4g | Fiber: 6g | Sodium: 310mg

Glycemic Index: Quinoa: Low (GI = 53) | Almonds: Low (GI = 15) | Mixed berries: Low (GI = 40)

Chia and Flax Seed Porridge with Coconut Milk and Blueberries

Prep: 5 minutes | **Cook:** 5 minutes | **Serves:** 2

Ingredients:

- 2 tbsp chia seeds (20g)
- 1 tbsp ground flax seeds (10g)
- 1 cup unsweetened coconut milk (240ml)
- 1 tbsp low carb sweetener (5g)
- 1/2 cup fresh blueberries (75g)

Instructions:

1. In a small saucepan, heat coconut milk and stir in chia seeds, flax seeds, and low carb sweetener. Simmer for 5 minutes until thickened.
2. Serve in bowls, topped with fresh blueberries.

Nutritional Facts (Per Serving): Calories: 400 | Carbohydrates: 14g | Protein: 18g | Fat: 17g | Sugars: 4g | Fiber: 10g | Sodium: 300mg

Glycemic Index: Chia seeds: Low (GI = 1) | Flax seeds: Low (GI = 1) | Blueberries: Low (GI = 53)

Pumpkin Spice Quinoa Porridge with Almond Milk

Prep: 5 minutes | Cook: 15 minutes | Serves: 2

Ingredients:

- 1/2 cup cooked quinoa (85g)
- 1 cup unsweetened almond milk (240ml)
- 1/4 cup pumpkin purée (60g)
- 1 tbsp chia seeds (10g)
- 1/2 tsp pumpkin spice (1g)
- 1 tbsp low carb sweetener (5g)

Instructions:

1. In a small pot, combine cooked quinoa, almond milk, pumpkin purée, chia seeds, pumpkin spice, and low carb sweetener.
2. Simmer on medium heat for 5-7 minutes until thickened.
3. Serve warm.

Nutritional Facts (Per Serving): Calories: 400 | Carbohydrates: 22g | Protein: 19g | Fat: 15g | Sugars: 3g | Fiber: 6g | Sodium: 300mg

Glycemic Index: Quinoa: Low (GI = 53) | Pumpkin: Low (GI = 51) | Almond milk: Low (GI = 30)

Flaxseed Porridge with Cinnamon and Chopped Pecans

Prep: 5 minutes | Cook: 5 minutes | Serves: 2

Ingredients:

- 2 tbsp ground flaxseeds (20g)
- 1 cup unsweetened almond milk (240ml)
- 1/2 tsp cinnamon (1g)
- 2 tbsp chopped pecans (30g)
- 1 tbsp low carb sweetener (5g)

Instructions:

1. Heat almond milk in a small saucepan and stir in ground flaxseeds, cinnamon, and low carb sweetener.
2. Simmer for 3-5 minutes until thickened.
3. Serve in bowls, topped with chopped pecans.

Nutritional Facts (Per Serving): Calories: 400 | Carbohydrates: 10g | Protein: 19g | Fat: 17g | Sugars: 2g | Fiber: 7g | Sodium: 300mg

Glycemic Index: Flaxseeds: Low (GI = 1) | Pecans: Low (GI = 15) | Almond milk: Low (GI = 30)

Buckwheat Porridge with Almonds and Raspberries

Prep: 5 minutes | Cook: 10 minutes | Serves: 2

Ingredients:

- 1/2 cup cooked buckwheat groats (85g)
- 1 cup unsweetened almond milk (240ml)
- 1 tbsp chopped almonds (15g)
- 1/2 cup fresh raspberries (75g)
- 1 tbsp low carb sweetener (5g)

Instructions:

1. In a small pot, combine cooked buckwheat groats, almond milk, and low carb sweetener.
2. Simmer for 5 minutes until thickened.
3. Serve in bowls, topped with chopped almonds and fresh raspberries.

Nutritional Facts (Per Serving): Calories: 400 | Carbohydrates: 20g | Protein: 18g | Fat: 16g | Sugars: 4g | Fiber: 6g | Sodium: 310mg

Glycemic Index: Buckwheat: Low (GI = 49) | Almonds: Low (GI = 15) | Raspberries: Low (GI = 32)

Almond Butter Couscous Porridge with Blueberries and Flaxseeds

Prep: 5 minutes | **Cook:** 10 minutes | **Serves:** 2

Ingredients:

- 1/2 cup couscous (85g)
- 1 cup unsweetened almond milk (240ml)
- 1 tbsp almond butter (16g)
- 1 tbsp ground flaxseeds (10g)
- 1/2 cup fresh blueberries (75g)
- 1 tbsp low carb sweetener (5g)

Instructions:

1. In a small pot, bring almond milk to a simmer, then stir in couscous. Cover and remove from heat. Let sit for 5 minutes until couscous is cooked.
2. Stir in almond butter, flaxseeds, and low carb sweetener.
3. Serve in bowls and top with fresh blueberries.

Nutritional Facts (Per Serving): Calories: 400 | Carbohydrates: 26g | Protein: 18g | Fat: 15g | Sugars: 3g | Fiber: 7g | Sodium: 300mg

Glycemic Index: Couscous: Medium (GI = 65) | Almond butter: Low (GI = 15) | Blueberries: Low (GI = 53)

Kale and Coconut Protein Bowl

Prep: 10 minutes | **Cook:** 10 minutes | **Serves:** 1

Ingredients:

- 1 cup chopped kale (30g)
- 2 tbsp unsweetened shredded coconut (16g)
- 1/2 cup cooked tofu cubes (100g)
- 1/2 tbsp olive oil (7ml)
- 1/2 tsp lemon juice (2.5ml)
- 1/4 tsp black pepper (1g)
- 1/8 tsp salt (0.5g)

Instructions:

1. In a pan, heat olive oil and sauté kale for 3–4 minutes.
2. Add tofu cubes and cook another 5 minutes.
3. Remove from heat, stir in lemon juice, shredded coconut, salt, and pepper.
4. Serve warm.

Nutritional Facts (Per Serving): Calories: 398 | Carbohydrates: 11g | Protein: 21g | Fat: 17g | Sugars: 2g | Fiber: 5g | Sodium: 350mg

Glycemic Index: Kale: 15 | Coconut: 45 | Tofu: 15

Blueberry Spinach Smoothie with Flaxseeds

Prep: 5 minutes | **Cook:** None | **Serves:** 1

Ingredients:

- 1/2 cup fresh blueberries (75g)
- 1/2 cup baby spinach (15g)
- 1 tbsp ground flaxseeds (10g)
- 1/2 cup unsweetened almond milk (120ml)
- 1/4 cup plain Greek yogurt (60g)
- 1/2 tsp cinnamon (1g)
- 1 tsp monk fruit sweetener (2g)

Instructions:

1. Blend all ingredients until smooth.
2. Serve chilled.

Nutritional Facts (Per Serving): Calories: 392 | Carbohydrates: 17g | Protein: 19g | Fat: 15g | Sugars: 5g | Fiber: 6g | Sodium: 300mg

Glycemic Index: Blueberries: 53 | Spinach: 15 | Flaxseeds: 1

Savory Greek Bowl with Eggs and Olives

Prep: 7 minutes | Cook: 10 minutes | Serves: 1

Ingredients:

- 2 large eggs (100g)
- 1/4 cup diced cucumber (50g)
- 1/4 cup chopped cherry tomatoes (50g)
- 2 tbsp diced Kalamata olives (15g)
- 1 tbsp crumbled feta cheese (15g)
- 1 tsp olive oil (5ml)
- 1/4 tsp black pepper (1g)
- 1/8 tsp salt (0.5g)

Instructions:

1. Hard-boil the eggs (9 minutes), peel and slice.
2. In a bowl, combine cucumber, tomatoes, olives, and feta.
3. Add sliced eggs on top, drizzle with olive oil, sprinkle salt and pepper.
4. Serve immediately.

Nutritional Facts (Per Serving): Calories: 395 | Carbohydrates: 10g | Protein: 21g | Fat: 18g | Sugars: 3g | Fiber: 3g | Sodium: 480mg

Glycemic Index: Eggs: 0 | Cucumber: 15 | Tomatoes: 30 | Olives: 15 | Feta: 0

Avocado and Chia Seed Smoothie

Prep: 5 minutes | Cook: None | Serves: 1

Ingredients:

- 1/2 avocado (70g)
- 1/2 cup unsweetened almond milk (120ml)
- 1 tbsp chia seeds (10g)
- 1/2 tsp vanilla extract (2.5ml)
- 1/2 tsp cinnamon (1.5g)
- 1 tsp monk fruit sweetener (2g)
- 3 ice cubes

Instructions:

1. Blend all ingredients together until smooth.
2. Serve immediately, chilled.

Nutritional Facts (Per Serving): Calories: 385 | Carbohydrates: 11g | Protein: 9g | Fat: 28g | Sugars: 1g | Fiber: 9g | Sodium: 180mg

Glycemic Index: Avocado: 15 | Chia seeds: 1 | Almond milk: 25

Zucchini and Egg Protein Bowl

Prep: 8 minutes | Cook: 12 minutes | Serves: 1

Ingredients:

- 1/2 cup shredded zucchini (60g)
- 2 large eggs (100g)
- 1/4 cup diced bell pepper (40g)
- 1 tbsp grated Parmesan cheese (7g)
- 1/2 tbsp olive oil (7ml)
- 1/4 tsp garlic powder (0.5g)
- 1/4 tsp black pepper (1g)
- 1/8 tsp salt (0.5g)

Instructions:

1. Heat olive oil in a skillet. Add zucchini and bell pepper. Sauté for 5 minutes.
2. Whisk eggs with garlic, salt, pepper, and parmesan.
3. Add eggs to the skillet and scramble until cooked through.
4. Serve in a bowl.

Nutritional Facts (Per Serving): Calories: 388 | Carbohydrates: 6g | Protein: 22g | Fat: 17g | Sugars: 2g | Fiber: 2g | Sodium: 430mg

Glycemic Index: Eggs: 0 | Zucchini: 15 | Bell pepper: 15 | Parmesan: 0

Strawberry Almond Breakfast Smoothie

Prep: 5 minutes | Cook: None | Serves: 1

Ingredients:

- 1/2 cup fresh strawberries (75g)
- 1 tbsp almond butter (16g)
- 1/4 cup Greek yogurt, plain (60g)
- 1/2 cup unsweetened soy milk (120ml)
- 1/2 tsp monk fruit sweetener (1g)
- 1/4 tsp cinnamon (0.5g)
- 2–3 ice cubes

Instructions:

1. Add all ingredients to a blender and blend until creamy.
2. Serve cold.

Nutritional Facts (Per Serving): Calories: 390 | Carbohydrates: 15g | Protein: 20g | Fat: 17g | Sugars: 5g | Fiber: 4g | Sodium: 270mg

Glycemic Index: Strawberries: 41 | Almond butter: 10 | Soy milk: 30

Cauliflower and Egg Power Bowl

Prep: 10 minutes | Cook: 15 minutes | Serves: 1

Ingredients:

- 1 cup riced cauliflower (100g)
- 2 large eggs (100g)
- 1/4 cup chopped spinach (15g)
- 1/4 tsp black pepper (1g)
- 1/8 tsp salt (0.5g)
- 1 tbsp grated cheddar cheese (15g)
- 1 tsp olive oil (5ml)
- 1/4 tsp smoked paprika (0.5g)

Instructions:

1. Heat olive oil in a skillet. Add cauliflower and paprika; cook for 5 minutes.
2. Stir in spinach and sauté 1–2 minutes.
3. In a separate pan, scramble eggs with salt and pepper.
4. Assemble in a bowl: cauliflower base, topped with eggs and cheese.

Nutritional Facts (Per Serving): Calories: 395 | Carbohydrates: 9g | Protein: 21g | Fat: 17g | Sugars: 2g | Fiber: 4g | Sodium: 440mg

Glycemic Index: Cauliflower: 15 | Eggs: 0 | Spinach: 15 | Cheddar: 0

Nutty Green Smoothie with Zucchini and Almonds

Prep: 5 minutes | Cook: None | Serves: 1

Ingredients:

- 1/2 cup raw zucchini, sliced (50g)
- 1 tbsp almond butter (16g)
- 1/4 small banana (25g)
- 1/2 cup unsweetened almond milk (120ml)
- 1 tbsp chia seeds (10g)
- 1/2 tsp cinnamon (1.5g)
- 1/2 tsp monk fruit sweetener (1g)

Instructions:

1. Blend all ingredients until smooth.
2. Serve immediately.

Nutritional Facts (Per Serving): Calories: 372 | Carbohydrates: 18g | Protein: 10g | Fat: 17g | Sugars: 5g | Fiber: 6g | Sodium: 220mg

Glycemic Index: Zucchini: 15 | Banana (small portion): 45 | Almond butter: 10 | Chia: 1

High-Protein Dishes to Stabilize Blood Sugar

Broccoli and Cheddar Scramble with Herbs

Prep: 5 minutes | **Cook:** 10 minutes | **Serves:** 2

Ingredients:

- 4 large eggs (200g)
- 1/2 cup steamed broccoli florets (75g)
- 1/4 cup shredded cheddar cheese (30g)
- 1 tbsp olive oil (15ml)
- 1 tbsp chopped fresh herbs (parsley, chives) (5g)
- 1/4 tsp black pepper (1g)
- 1/8 tsp salt (0.5g)

Instructions:

1. Heat oil, add broccoli, cook 1 min.
2. Whisk eggs with herbs, salt, pepper. Pour in.
3. Stir 3–4 min until softly scrambled.
4. Add cheese, melt. Serve.

Nutritional Facts (Per Serving): Calories: 400 | Carbohydrates: 6g | Protein: 20g | Fat: 17g | Sugars: 2g | Fiber: 2g | Sodium: 390mg

Glycemic Index: Eggs: Negligible GI | Broccoli: Low (GI = 15) | Cheddar: Low (GI = 0)

Soft-Boiled Eggs with Sautéed Kale and Mushrooms

Prep: 5 minutes | **Cook:** 10 minutes | **Serves:** 2

Ingredients:

- 4 large eggs (200g)
- 1 cup chopped kale (30g)
- 1 cup sliced mushrooms (100g)
- 1 tbsp olive oil (15ml)
- 1/2 tsp lemon juice (2.5ml)
- 1/4 tsp black pepper (1g)
- 1/8 tsp salt (0.5g)

Instructions:

1. Boil eggs 6 min, peel.
2. Sauté kale & mushrooms in oil 3–4 min.
3. Add lemon juice, salt, pepper.
4. Serve with eggs.

Nutritional Facts (Per Serving): Calories: 400 | Carbohydrates: 8g | Protein: 20g | Fat: 17g | Sugars: 2g | Fiber: 3g | Sodium: 320mg

Glycemic Index: Eggs: Negligible GI | Kale: Low (GI = 15) | Mushrooms: Low (GI = 15)

Spinach and Feta Stuffed Chicken Breasts

Prep: 10 minutes | **Cook:** 20 minutes | **Serves:** 2

Ingredients:

- 2 boneless, skinless chicken breasts (300g)
- 1 cup fresh spinach, chopped (30g)
- 1/4 cup crumbled feta cheese (60g)
- 1 tbsp olive oil (15ml)
- 1/4 tsp black pepper (1g)
- 1/8 tsp salt (0.5g)

Instructions:

1. Preheat oven to 375°F (190°C).
2. Butterfly the chicken breasts and stuff with spinach and feta cheese. Secure with toothpicks.
3. Heat olive oil in an oven-safe skillet over medium heat and sear the chicken on both sides for 2-3 minutes.
4. Transfer skillet to the oven and bake for 15-18 minutes until the chicken is cooked through.
5. Remove toothpicks and serve.

Nutritional Facts (Per Serving): Calories: 400 | Carbohydrates: 4g | Protein: 22g | Fat: 15g | Sugars: 1g | Fiber: 1g | Sodium: 380mg

Glycemic Index: Chicken: Negligible GI | Spinach: Low (GI = 15) | Feta: Low (GI = 0)

Egg White and Turkey Sausage Scramble

Prep: 5 minutes | Cook: 10 minutes | Serves: 2

Ingredients:

- 6 large egg whites (180g)
- 4 oz turkey sausage, crumbled (115g)
- 1 tbsp olive oil (15ml)
- 1/4 cup diced bell peppers (40g)
- 1/4 tsp black pepper (1g)
- 1/8 tsp salt (0.5g)

Instructions:

1. Heat olive oil in a pan over medium heat. Add turkey sausage and cook for 5 minutes until browned.
2. Add diced bell peppers and cook for 2 minutes until softened.
3. Pour in egg whites, season with black pepper and salt, and scramble until fully cooked.

Nutritional Facts (Per Serving): Calories: 400 | Carbohydrates: 5g | Protein: 22g | Fat: 14g | Sugars: 2g | Fiber: 1g | Sodium: 400mg

Glycemic Index: Egg whites: Negligible GI | Bell peppers: Low (GI = 15) | Turkey sausage: Low (GI = 28)

Grilled Chicken Salad with Avocado and Quinoa

Prep: 10 minutes | Cook: 15 minutes | Serves: 2

Ingredients:

- 2 grilled chicken breasts (300g)
- 1 small avocado, sliced (120g)
- 1/2 cup cooked quinoa (85g)
- 2 cups mixed greens (60g)
- 1 tbsp olive oil (15ml)
- 1 tbsp lemon juice (15ml)
- 1/4 tsp black pepper (1g)
- 1/8 tsp salt (0.5g)

Instructions:

1. In a large bowl, combine mixed greens, quinoa, and sliced avocado.
2. Slice the grilled chicken and place on top of the salad.
3. Drizzle with olive oil, lemon juice, and season with black pepper and salt. Toss lightly and serve.

Nutritional Facts (Per Serving): Calories: 400 | Carbohydrates: 18g | Protein: 22g | Fat: 17g | Sugars: 2g | Fiber: 7g | Sodium: 350mg

Glycemic Index: Chicken: Negligible GI | Quinoa: Low (GI = 53) | Avocado: Low (GI = 15)

Beef and Broccoli Stir-Fry with Sesame Seeds

Prep: 10 minutes | Cook: 15 minutes | Serves: 2

Ingredients:

- 8 oz beef sirloin, sliced thinly (225g)
- 2 cups broccoli florets (150g)
- 1 tbsp olive oil (15ml)
- 2 tbsp low-sodium soy sauce (30ml)
- 1 tbsp sesame oil (15ml)
- 1 tsp sesame seeds (5g)
- 1 tsp minced garlic (5g)
- 1 tsp minced ginger (5g)
- 1/4 tsp black pepper (1g)

Instructions:

1. Heat olive oil in a large pan over medium heat. Add sliced beef and cook for 5 minutes until browned.
2. Add minced garlic, ginger, and broccoli florets to the pan. Stir-fry for 4-5 minutes until broccoli is tender.
3. Pour in soy sauce and sesame oil, stir well. Cook for 2 minutes more.
4. Serve topped with sesame seeds.

Nutritional Facts (Per Serving): Calories: 400 | Carbohydrates: 10g | Protein: 22g | Fat: 16g | Sugars: 3g | Fiber: 3g | Sodium: 450mg

Glycemic Index: Beef: Negligible GI | Broccoli: Low (GI = 15) | Sesame seeds: Low (GI = 35)

Turkey and Spinach Meatballs with Zucchini Noodles

Prep: 10 minutes | Cook: 20 minutes | Serves: 2

Ingredients:

- 8 oz ground turkey (225g)
- 1 cup fresh spinach, chopped (30g)
- 1 egg (50g)
- 1/4 cup almond flour (30g)
- 1 tbsp olive oil (15ml)
- 2 medium zucchinis, spiralized (200g)
- 1/4 tsp black pepper (1g)
- 1/8 tsp salt (0.5g)

Instructions:

1. Preheat oven to 375°F (190°C). In a bowl, mix ground turkey, spinach, egg, almond flour, black pepper, and salt. Form into small meatballs.
2. Place meatballs on a baking sheet and bake for 15-18 minutes until cooked through.
3. While the meatballs bake, heat olive oil in a pan and sauté zucchini noodles for 3-4 minutes until tender.
4. Serve meatballs over zucchini noodles.

Nutritional Facts (Per Serving): Calories: 400 | Carbohydrates: 12g | Protein: 22g | Fat: 15g | Sugars: 3g | Fiber: 4g | Sodium: 400mg

Glycemic Index: Turkey: Negligible GI | Zucchini: Low (GI = 15) | Almond flour: Low (GI = 15)

Egg and Spinach Breakfast Muffins with Turkey Bacon

Prep: 10 minutes | Cook: 20 minutes | Serves: 2

Ingredients:

- 6 large eggs (300g)
- 1 cup fresh spinach, chopped (30g)
- 4 slices turkey bacon, cooked and chopped (120g)
- 1/4 cup shredded cheddar cheese (30g)
- 1 tbsp olive oil (15ml)
- 1/4 tsp black pepper (1g)
- 1/8 tsp salt (0.5g)

Instructions:

1. Preheat oven to 350°F (175°C). Grease a muffin tin with olive oil.
2. In a bowl, whisk eggs with black pepper and salt. Stir in chopped spinach, turkey bacon, and cheddar cheese.
3. Pour the mixture into the muffin tin and bake for 18-20 minutes until set.
4. Serve warm.

Nutritional Facts (Per Serving): Calories: 400 | Carbohydrates: 5g | Protein: 22g | Fat: 17g | Sugars: 1g | Fiber: 1g | Sodium: 450mg

Glycemic Index: Eggs: Negligible GI | Spinach: Low (GI = 15) | Turkey bacon: Low (GI = 30)

Chicken and Chickpea Salad with Avocado and Lime

Prep: 10 minutes | Cook: None | Serves: 2

Ingredients:

- 6 oz cooked chicken breast, chopped (170g)
- 1/2 cup cooked chickpeas (85g)
- 1 small avocado, diced (120g)
- 1 tbsp olive oil (15ml)
- 1 tbsp lime juice (15ml)
- 1 cup mixed greens (30g)
- 1/4 tsp black pepper (1g)
- 1/8 tsp salt (0.5g)

Instructions:

1. In a bowl, combine cooked chicken, chickpeas, avocado, and mixed greens.
2. Drizzle with olive oil and lime juice. Season with black pepper and salt.
3. Toss lightly and serve chilled.

Nutritional Facts (Per Serving): Calories: 400 | Carbohydrates: 20g | Protein: 22g | Fat: 17g | Sugars: 2g | Fiber: 8g | Sodium: 350mg

Glycemic Index: Chicken: Negligible GI | Chickpeas: Low (GI = 28) | Avocado: Low (GI = 15)

Grilled Steak with Roasted Vegetables and Quinoa

Prep: 15 minutes | Cook: 25 minutes | Serves: 2

Ingredients:

- 8 oz steak (225g)
- 1 cup diced zucchini (150g)
- 1 cup diced bell peppers (150g)
- 1 tbsp olive oil (15ml)
- 1/2 cup cooked quinoa (85g)
- 1 tbsp balsamic vinegar (15ml)
- 1/4 tsp black pepper (1g)
- 1/8 tsp salt (0.5g)

Instructions:

1. Preheat grill to medium-high heat. Season the steak with black pepper and salt, and grill for 4-5 minutes per side, or until desired doneness.
2. Toss zucchini and bell peppers with olive oil, then roast at 400°F (200°C) for 20 minutes until tender.
3. Serve the steak with roasted vegetables and quinoa, drizzling balsamic vinegar on top.

Nutritional Facts (Per Serving): Calories: 400 | Carbohydrates: 20g | Protein: 22g | Fat: 15g | Sugars: 3g | Fiber: 4g | Sodium: 400mg

Glycemic Index: Steak: Negligible GI | Quinoa: Low (GI = 53) | Zucchini: Low (GI = 15) | Bell peppers: Low (GI = 15)

Turkey and Black Bean Chili with Avocado

Prep: 10 minutes | Cook: 25 minutes | Serves: 2

Ingredients:

- 8 oz ground turkey (225g)
- 1/2 cup cooked black beans (85g)
- 1 small avocado, diced (120g)
- 1 cup diced tomatoes (150g)
- 1 tbsp olive oil (15ml)
- 1 tsp chili powder (5g)
- 1/2 tsp cumin (2g)
- 1/4 tsp black pepper (1g)
- 1/8 tsp salt (0.5g)

Instructions:

1. Heat olive oil in a large pan over medium heat. Add ground turkey and cook until browned, about 5-7 minutes.
2. Stir in black beans, diced tomatoes, chili powder, cumin, black pepper, and salt. Simmer for 15 minutes.
3. Serve topped with diced avocado.

Nutritional Facts (Per Serving): Calories: 400 | Carbohydrates: 22g | Protein: 22g | Fat: 17g | Sugars: 3g | Fiber: 9g | Sodium: 450mg

Glycemic Index: Turkey: Negligible GI | Black beans: Low (GI = 30) | Avocado: Low (GI = 15)

Baked Chicken Thighs with Roasted Cauliflower

Prep: 10 minutes | Cook: 25 minutes | Serves: 2

Ingredients:

- 4 boneless, skinless chicken thighs (300g)
- 2 cups cauliflower florets (200g)
- 1 tbsp olive oil (15ml)
- 1 tsp paprika (5g)
- 1/4 tsp black pepper (1g)
- 1/8 tsp salt (0.5g)

Instructions:

1. Preheat oven to 400°F (200°C).
2. Season chicken thighs with paprika, black pepper, and salt.
3. Toss cauliflower florets in olive oil, black pepper, and salt.
4. Place chicken and cauliflower on a baking sheet and roast for 20-25 minutes until chicken is fully cooked and cauliflower is tender.
5. Serve warm.

Nutritional Facts (Per Serving): Calories: 400 | Carbohydrates: 8g | Protein: 22g | Fat: 15g | Sugars: 2g | Fiber: 4g | Sodium: 450mg

Glycemic Index: Chicken: Negligible GI | Cauliflower: Low (GI = 15)

Low-Carb Cottage Cheese and Spinach Pancakes

Prep: 5 minutes | **Cook:** 10 minutes | **Serves:** 2

Ingredients:

- 1/2 cup cottage cheese (120g)
- 1/2 cup baby spinach, chopped (30g)
- 2 large eggs (100g)
- 1/4 cup almond flour (30g)
- 1 tsp olive oil (5ml)
- 1/4 tsp black pepper (1g)
- 1/8 tsp salt (0.5g)

Instructions:

1. In a bowl, mix cottage cheese, chopped spinach, eggs, almond flour, black pepper, and salt.
2. Heat olive oil in a non-stick pan over medium heat.
3. Spoon batter into the pan to form small pancakes and cook for 3-4 minutes on each side until golden brown.
4. Serve warm.

Nutritional Facts (Per Serving): Calories: 400 | Carbohydrates: 9g | Protein: 20g | Fat: 15g | Sugars: 2g | Fiber: 3g | Sodium: 350mg

Glycemic Index: Cottage cheese: Low (GI = 27) | Spinach: Low (GI = 15) | Almond flour: Low (GI = 15)

Lentil and Quinoa Stew with Turkey Sausage

Prep: 10 minutes | **Cook:** 25 minutes | **Serves:** 2

Ingredients:

- 4 oz turkey sausage, sliced (115g)
- 1/2 cup cooked lentils (85g)
- 1/2 cup cooked quinoa (85g)
- 1 cup diced tomatoes (150g)
- 1 tbsp olive oil (15ml)
- 1 tsp cumin (5g)
- 1/2 tsp paprika (2g)
- 1/4 tsp black pepper (1g)
- 1/8 tsp salt (0.5g)

Instructions:

1. Heat olive oil in a large pot over medium heat. Add turkey sausage and cook for 5 minutes until browned.
2. Add diced tomatoes, cooked lentils, cooked quinoa, cumin, paprika, black pepper, and salt.
3. Simmer for 15 minutes until the stew thickens.
4. Serve warm.

Nutritional Facts (Per Serving): Calories: 400 | Carbohydrates: 24g | Protein: 21g | Fat: 15g | Sugars: 3g | Fiber: 7g | Sodium: 400mg

Glycemic Index: Lentils: Low (GI = 32) | Quinoa: Low (GI = 53) | Turkey sausage: Low (GI = 28)

Turkey Lettuce Wraps with Avocado and Cucumber

Prep: 10 minutes | **Cook:** 5 minutes | **Serves:** 2

Ingredients:

- 6 oz ground turkey (170g)
- 1 small avocado, sliced (120g)
- 1/2 cucumber, sliced (75g)
- 1 tbsp olive oil (15ml)
- 1/8 tsp salt (0.5g)
- 1 tbsp lime juice (15ml)
- 8 large lettuce leaves (60g)
- 1/4 tsp black pepper (1g)

Instructions:

1. Heat olive oil in a pan over medium heat. Add ground turkey and cook for 5-7 minutes until browned, seasoning with black pepper and salt.
2. Lay the lettuce leaves flat and fill with cooked turkey, sliced avocado, and cucumber.
3. Drizzle with lime juice and roll into wraps. Serve immediately.

Nutritional Facts (Per Serving): Calories: 400 | Carbohydrates: 10g | Protein: 22g | Fat: 17g | Sugars: 2g | Fiber: 5g | Sodium: 350mg

Glycemic Index: Turkey: Negligible GI | Avocado: Low (GI = 15) | Cucumber: Low (GI = 15) | Lettuce: Low (GI = 15)

Grilled Chicken Bowl with Spinach and Tahini

Prep: 10 minutes | **Cook:** 12 minutes | **Serves:** 1

Ingredients:

- 6 oz chicken breast, grilled and sliced (170g)
- 1 cup baby spinach (30g)
- 1 tbsp tahini (15g)
- 1/2 tbsp olive oil (7ml)
- 1 tbsp lemon juice (15ml)
- 1/4 tsp cumin (0.5g)
- 1/4 tsp black pepper (1g)
- 1/8 tsp salt (0.5g)

Instructions:

1. Grill the chicken breast until fully cooked, then slice.
2. In a bowl, toss spinach with olive oil, lemon juice, cumin, salt, and pepper.
3. Add grilled chicken on top, drizzle with tahini.
4. Serve immediately.

Nutritional Facts (Per Serving): Calories: 398 | Carbohydrates: 6g | Protein: 25g | Fat: 18g | Sugar: 1g | Fiber: 2g | Sodium: 410mg

Glycemic Index: Chicken: 0 | Spinach: 15 | Tahini: 35

Lentil and Turkey Mini Patties

Prep: 10 minutes | **Cook:** 15 minutes | **Serves:** 2

Ingredients:

- 3 oz lean ground turkey (85g)
- 1/4 cup cooked green lentils (60g)
- 1 tbsp chopped parsley (5g)
- 1/4 tsp garlic powder (0.5g)
- 1/4 tsp paprika (0.5g)
- 1/4 tsp salt (0.5g)
- 1/8 tsp black pepper (0.5g)
- 1/2 tbsp olive oil (7ml)

Instructions:

1. Mix turkey, lentils, parsley, and spices in a bowl.
2. Form 2 small patties.
3. Heat olive oil in a non-stick pan and cook patties for 5–6 minutes per side.
4. Serve warm with greens or yogurt dip.

Nutritional Facts (Per Serving): Calories: 395 | Carbohydrates: 12g | Protein: 24g | Fat: 17g | Sugar: 2g | Fiber: 4g | Sodium: 430mg

Glycemic Index: Turkey: 0 | Lentils: 32 | Olive oil: 0

Egg and Cottage Cheese Bake with Broccoli

Prep: 10 minutes | **Cook:** 20 minutes | **Serves:** 1

Ingredients:

- 2 large eggs (100g)
- 1/2 cup low-fat cottage cheese (120g)
- 1/2 cup steamed broccoli florets (75g)
- 1 tbsp grated Parmesan (7g)
- 1/4 tsp black pepper (1g)
- 1/8 tsp salt (0.5g)

Instructions:

1. Preheat oven to 375°F (190°C).
2. In a bowl, whisk eggs with salt and pepper.
3. Add cottage cheese and broccoli, mix gently.
4. Pour into a greased ramekin, top with Parmesan.
5. Bake for 18–20 minutes or until set. Serve warm.

Nutritional Facts (Per Serving): Calories: 385 | Carbohydrates: 7g | Protein: 24g | Fat: 17g | Sugar: 2g | Fiber: 2g | Sodium: 400mg

Glycemic Index: Eggs: 0 | Broccoli: 15 | Cottage cheese: 30

Beef and Zucchini Skillet

Prep: 8 minutes | Cook: 15 minutes | Serves: 1

Ingredients:

- 4 oz lean ground beef (115g)
- 1/2 cup chopped zucchini (60g)
- 1/4 cup diced tomatoes (50g)
- 1/2 tbsp olive oil (7ml)
- 1/4 tsp dried oregano (0.5g)
- 1/4 tsp black pepper (1g)
- 1/8 tsp salt (0.5g)

Instructions:

1. Heat olive oil in a skillet. Add ground beef and cook for 5–6 minutes.
2. Add zucchini, tomatoes, and spices. Cook for another 7–8 minutes.
3. Serve hot with fresh herbs if desired.

Nutritional Facts (Per Serving): Calories: 400 | Carbohydrates: 8g | Protein: 25g | Fat: 18g | Sugar: 3g | Fiber: 2g | Sodium: 430mg

Glycemic Index: Beef: 0 | Zucchini: 15 | Tomatoes: 30

Baked Tofu Nuggets with Mustard Dip

Prep: 10 minutes | Cook: 20 minutes | Serves: 1

Ingredients:

- 3/4 cup firm tofu, cubed (120g)
- 1 tbsp almond flour (10g)
- 1/4 tsp garlic powder (0.5g)
- 1/2 tsp Dijon mustard (2g)
- 1/4 tsp paprika (0.5g)
- 1/8 tsp salt (0.5g)
- 1/2 tbsp olive oil (7ml)
- 1 tbsp plain Greek yogurt (20g)

Instructions:

1. Preheat oven to 375°F (190°C).
2. Toss tofu cubes with almond flour, spices, and olive oil.
3. Arrange on baking sheet and bake for 20 minutes, flipping halfway.
4. Mix yogurt and mustard for dipping. Serve together.

Nutritional Facts (Per Serving): Calories: 390 | Carbohydrates: 9g | Protein: 23g | Fat: 17g | Sugar: 2g | Fiber: 3g | Sodium: 320mg

Glycemic Index: Tofu: 15 | Almond flour: 10 | Yogurt: 10 | Mustard: 35

Egg, Kale and Turkey Stir-Fry

Prep: 7 minutes | Cook: 10 minutes | Serves: 1

Ingredients:

- 1 large egg (50g)
- 2 oz cooked turkey breast, chopped (60g)
- 1 cup kale, chopped (30g)
- 1/2 tbsp olive oil (7ml)
- 1/4 tsp turmeric (0.5g)
- 1/4 tsp black pepper (1g)
- 1/8 tsp salt (0.5g)

Instructions:

1. Heat olive oil in a skillet. Add turkey and kale; sauté for 3–4 minutes.
2. Crack in the egg and scramble with turmeric, salt, and pepper.
3. Cook until egg is set. Serve immediately.

Nutritional Facts (Per Serving): Calories: 382 | Carbohydrates: 4g | Protein: 24g | Fat: 17g | Sugar: 1g | Fiber: 2g | Sodium: 390mg

Glycemic Index: Egg: 0 | Kale: 15 | Turkey: 0

Cottage Cheese Omelet with Herbs

Prep: 5 minutes | Cook: 10 minutes | Serves: 1

Ingredients:

- 2 large eggs (100g)
- 1/2 cup low-fat cottage cheese (100g)
- 1 tbsp chopped fresh parsley (4g)
- 1/4 tsp black pepper (1g)
- 1/8 tsp salt (0.5g)
- 1/2 tbsp olive oil (7ml)

Instructions:

1. In a bowl, whisk eggs with salt, pepper, and parsley.
2. Stir in cottage cheese.
3. Heat olive oil in a non-stick skillet. Pour in egg mixture.
4. Cook on medium heat for 4–5 minutes until set. Fold and serve.

Nutritional Facts (Per Serving): Calories: 385 | Carbohydrates: 4g | Protein: 23g | Fat: 17g | Sugar: 2g | Fiber: 1g | Sodium: 420mg

Glycemic Index: Eggs: 0 | Cottage cheese: 30 | Parsley: 15

Turkey and Cabbage Stir-Fry

Prep: 7 minutes | Cook: 12 minutes | Serves: 1

Ingredients:

- 4 oz turkey breast, chopped (115g)
- 1 cup shredded white cabbage (70g)
- 1/2 tbsp olive oil (7ml)
- 1/4 tsp garlic powder (0.5g)
- 1/4 tsp black pepper (1g)
- 1/8 tsp salt (0.5g)

Instructions:

1. Heat olive oil in a skillet.
2. Add turkey, garlic powder, salt, and pepper; sauté for 5 minutes.
3. Stir in cabbage and cook another 5–6 minutes until soft.
4. Serve warm.

Nutritional Facts (Per Serving): Calories: 390 | Carbohydrates: 7g | Protein: 25g | Fat: 17g | Sugar: 2g | Fiber: 3g | Sodium: 410mg

Glycemic Index: Turkey: 0 | Cabbage: 15

Tuna Salad Bowl with Boiled Egg and Greens

Prep: 10 minutes | Cook: 8 minutes | Serves: 1

Ingredients:

- 1 boiled egg (50g)
- 1/2 can tuna in water, drained (70g)
- 1/2 cup cucumber slices (50g)
- 1/2 cup mixed greens (20g)
- 1 tbsp olive oil (15ml)
- 1 tsp lemon juice (5ml)
- 1/4 tsp mustard (1g)
- 1/8 tsp salt (0.5g)
- 1/4 tsp black pepper (1g)

Instructions:

1. Boil the egg, peel and slice.
2. In a bowl, combine tuna, cucumber, greens, and egg.
3. Mix olive oil, lemon juice, mustard, salt, and pepper for dressing.
4. Drizzle over salad and serve.

Nutritional Facts (Per Serving): Calories: 395 | Carbohydrates: 5g | Protein: 24g | Fat: 18g | Sugar: 1g | Fiber: 2g | Sodium: 440mg

Glycemic Index: Tuna: 0 | Egg: 0 | Cucumber: 15 | Greens: 15

Weekend Brunch Ideas

Crustless Veggie Quiche with Bell Peppers and Onions

Prep: 10 minutes | Cook: 25 minutes | Serves: 2

Ingredients:

- 4 large eggs (200g)
- 1/2 cup diced bell peppers (75g)
- 1/2 cup diced onions (75g)
- 1 tbsp olive oil (15ml)
- 1/4 cup shredded cheddar cheese (30g)
- 1/4 tsp black pepper (1g)
- 1/8 tsp salt (0.5g)

Instructions:

1. Preheat oven to 375°F (190°C).
2. Heat olive oil in a pan over medium heat and sauté bell peppers and onions for 5 minutes until softened.
3. In a bowl, whisk eggs, black pepper, salt, and shredded cheddar. Stir in sautéed vegetables.
4. Pour mixture into a greased baking dish and bake for 20-25 minutes until set. Serve warm.

Nutritional Facts (Per Serving): Calories: 400 | Carbohydrates: 8g | Protein: 20g | Fat: 17g | Sugars: 3g | Fiber: 2g | Sodium: 400mg

Glycemic Index: Eggs: Negligible GI | Bell peppers: Low (GI = 15) | Onions: Low (GI = 10)

Zucchini and Egg Casserole with Feta and Oregano

Prep: 10 minutes | Cook: 25 minutes | Serves: 2

Ingredients:

- 4 large eggs (200g)
- 1 cup grated zucchini (150g)
- 1/4 cup crumbled feta cheese (60g)
- 1 tbsp olive oil (15ml)
- 1 tsp dried oregano (1g)
- 1/4 tsp black pepper (1g)
- 1/8 tsp salt (0.5g)

Instructions:

1. Preheat oven to 350°F (175°C).
2. In a bowl, mix grated zucchini, crumbled feta, eggs, oregano, black pepper, and salt.
3. Grease a baking dish with olive oil, pour the mixture into the dish, and bake for 20-25 minutes until golden and set.
4. Serve warm.

Nutritional Facts (Per Serving): Calories: 400 | Carbohydrates: 7g | Protein: 20g | Fat: 16g | Sugars: 2g | Fiber: 2g | Sodium: 450mg

Glycemic Index: Zucchini: Low (GI = 15) | Feta: Low (GI = 15)

Mushroom and Asparagus Egg Bake

Prep: 10 minutes | Cook: 25 minutes | Serves: 2

Ingredients:

- 4 large eggs (200g)
- 1 cup sliced mushrooms (100g)
- 1 cup chopped asparagus (100g)
- 1 tbsp olive oil (15ml)
- 1/4 cup shredded mozzarella cheese (30g)
- 1/4 tsp black pepper (1g)
- 1/8 tsp salt (0.5g)

Instructions:

1. Preheat oven to 375°F (190°C).
2. Heat olive oil in a pan over medium heat and sauté mushrooms and asparagus for 5 minutes until softened.
3. In a bowl, whisk eggs, black pepper, salt, and mozzarella cheese. Stir in sautéed vegetables.
4. Pour mixture into a greased baking dish and bake for 20-25 minutes until set.
5. Serve warm.

Nutritional Facts (Per Serving): Calories: 400 | Carbohydrates: 6g | Protein: 22g | Fat: 17g | Sugars: 2g | Fiber: 2g | Sodium: 400mg

Glycemic Index: Mushrooms: Low (GI = 15) | Asparagus: Low (GI = 15) | Eggs: Negligible GI

Cauliflower Rice Stir-Fry with Scrambled Eggs and Garlic

Prep: 10 minutes | Cook: 10 minutes | Serves: 2

Ingredients:

- 2 cups cauliflower rice (200g)
- 4 large eggs (200g)
- 1 tbsp olive oil (15ml)
- 2 garlic cloves, minced (6g)
- 1/4 tsp black pepper (1g)
- 1/8 tsp salt (0.5g)
- 1 tbsp soy sauce (15ml)

Instructions:

1. Heat olive oil in a pan over medium heat. Add minced garlic and sauté for 1 minute.
2. Stir-fry cauliflower rice for 5 minutes until tender.
3. Push the cauliflower to one side of the pan and scramble the eggs on the other side.
4. Mix everything together, season with black pepper, salt, and soy sauce. Serve warm.

Nutritional Facts (Per Serving): Calories: 400 | Carbohydrates: 9g | Protein: 20g | Fat: 17g | Sugars: 2g | Fiber: 4g | Sodium: 450mg

Glycemic Index: Cauliflower: Low (GI = 15) | Eggs: Negligible GI | Garlic: Low (GI = 10)

Almond Flour Pancakes with Blueberry Compote

Prep: 10 minutes | Cook: 10 minutes | Serves: 2

Ingredients:

- 1/2 cup almond flour (60g)
- 2 large eggs (100g)
- 1 tbsp olive oil (15ml)
- 1 tbsp low carb sweetener (5g)
- 1/4 tsp baking powder (1g)
- 1/2 cup fresh blueberries (75g)
- 1 tsp lemon juice (5ml)

Instructions:

1. In a bowl, whisk almond flour, eggs, olive oil, low carb sweetener, and baking powder to form a batter.
2. Heat a non-stick pan over medium heat and pour batter to form small pancakes. Cook for 2-3 minutes on each side.
3. For the compote, simmer blueberries with lemon juice over low heat for 5 minutes.
4. Serve pancakes topped with blueberry compote.

Nutritional Information (Per Serving): Calories: 400 | Carbohydrates: 14g | Protein: 20g | Fat: 17g | Sugars: 4g | Fiber: 5g | Sodium: 300mg

Glycemic Index: Almond flour: Low (GI = 15) | Blueberries: Low (GI = 53)

Coconut Flour Waffles with Cinnamon and Almond Butter

Prep: 10 minutes | Cook: 10 minutes | Serves: 2

Ingredients:

- 1/4 cup coconut flour (30g)
- 4 large eggs (200g)
- 1 tbsp olive oil (15ml)
- 1 tbsp almond butter (16g)
- 1/2 tsp ground cinnamon (1g)
- 1/4 tsp baking powder (1g)
- 1 tbsp low carb sweetener (5g)

Instructions:

1. In a bowl, whisk coconut flour, eggs, olive oil, almond butter, cinnamon, baking powder, and low carb sweetener.
2. Preheat a waffle iron and pour the batter to cook waffles for 3-4 minutes until golden brown.
3. Serve warm, drizzled with extra almond butter if desired.

Nutritional Facts (Per Serving): Calories: 400 | Carbohydrates: 11g | Protein: 19g | Fat: 16g | Sugars: 2g | Fiber: 6g | Sodium: 350mg

Glycemic Index: Coconut flour: Low (GI = 51) | Almond butter: Low (GI = 15) | Cinnamon: Low (GI = 5)

Keto Pumpkin Pancakes with Pecans

Prep: 10 minutes | Cook: 10 minutes | Serves: 2

Ingredients:

- 1/2 cup almond flour (60g)
- 1/4 cup pumpkin purée (60g)
- 2 large eggs (100g)
- 1 tbsp olive oil (15ml)
- 1 tbsp low carb sweetener (5g)
- 1/2 tsp ground cinnamon (1g)
- 1/4 cup chopped pecans (30g)

Instructions:

1. In a bowl, whisk almond flour, pumpkin purée, eggs, olive oil, low carb sweetener, and cinnamon until smooth.
2. Heat a non-stick pan over medium heat and cook pancakes for 2-3 minutes on each side until golden brown.
3. Serve topped with chopped pecans.

Nutritional Facts (Per Serving): Calories: 400 | Carbohydrates: 11g | Protein: 20g | Fat: 17g | Sugars: 3g | Fiber: 5g | Sodium: 350mg

Glycemic Index: Almond flour: Low (GI = 15) | Pumpkin: Low (GI = 51) | Pecans: Low (GI = 15)

Low-Carb Zucchini Fritters with Poached Eggs

Prep: 10 minutes | Cook: 15 minutes | Serves: 2

Ingredients:

- 2 medium zucchinis, grated (200g)
- 1/4 cup almond flour (30g)
- 2 large eggs (for poaching) (100g)
- 1 large egg, beaten (50g)
- 1 tbsp olive oil (15ml)
- 1/4 tsp black pepper (1g)
- 1/8 tsp salt (0.5g)

Instructions:

1. Grate zucchini and squeeze out excess moisture. Mix with almond flour, beaten egg, black pepper, and salt.
2. Heat olive oil in a pan and form the mixture into small fritters. Cook for 3 minutes on each side until golden brown.
3. Poach the eggs in simmering water for 3-4 minutes.
4. Serve fritters topped with poached eggs.

Nutritional Facts (Per Serving): Calories: 400 | Carbohydrates: 9g | Protein: 19g | Fat: 17g | Sugars: 2g | Fiber: 4g | Sodium: 320mg

Glycemic Index: Zucchini: Low (GI = 15) | Almond flour: Low (GI = 15)

Almond Flour Crepes with Ricotta and Spinach

Prep: 10 minutes | Cook: 10 minutes | Serves: 2

Ingredients:

- 1/2 cup almond flour (60g)
- 2 large eggs (100g)
- 1/4 cup unsweetened almond milk (60ml)
- 1/2 cup ricotta cheese (120g)
- 1 cup fresh spinach, chopped (30g)
- 1 tbsp olive oil (15ml)
- 1/4 tsp black pepper (1g)
- 1/8 tsp salt (0.5g)

Instructions:

1. In a bowl, whisk almond flour, eggs, almond milk, black pepper, and salt to form a crepe batter.
2. Heat olive oil in a non-stick pan and cook thin crepes for 1-2 minutes on each side.
3. Sauté spinach for 2 minutes, then mix with ricotta.
4. Fill the crepes with the ricotta-spinach mixture.

Nutritional Facts (Per Serving): Calories: 400 | Carbohydrates: 10g | Protein: 21g | Fat: 17g | Sugars: 2g | Fiber: 4g | Sodium: 340mg

Glycemic Index: Almond flour: Low (GI = 15) | Ricotta: Low (GI = 27) | Spinach: Low (GI = 15)

Low-Carb Pizzas with Turkey and Spinach

Prep: 10 minutes | Cook: 15 minutes | Serves: 2

Ingredients:

- 1/2 lb ground turkey (225g)
- 2 low-carb pizza crusts (100g each)
- 1 cup baby spinach, chopped (30g)
- 1/4 cup shredded mozzarella cheese (30g)
- 1 tbsp olive oil (15ml)
- 1/4 tsp black pepper (1g)
- 1/8 tsp salt (0.5g)

Instructions:

1. Preheat oven to 400°F (200°C).
2. In a pan, heat olive oil over medium heat, add ground turkey, and cook for 5 minutes until browned. Season with black pepper and salt.
3. Spread cooked turkey and chopped spinach evenly over the low-carb pizza crusts.
4. Top with mozzarella and bake 8-10 minutes until melted and crispy.

Nutritional Facts (Per Serving): Calories: 400 | Carbohydrates: 10g | Protein: 22g | Fat: 16g | Sugars: 2g | Fiber: 3g | Sodium: 400mg

Glycemic Index: Low-carb pizza crust: Low (GI = 15) | Turkey: Negligible GI | Spinach: Low (GI = 15)

Eggplant Breakfast Pizza with Scrambled Eggs and Parmesan

Prep: 10 minutes | Cook: 15 minutes | Serves: 2

Ingredients:

- 1 medium eggplant, sliced (200g)
- 4 large eggs (200g)
- 1/4 cup grated Parmesan cheese (30g)
- 1 tbsp olive oil (15ml)
- 1/4 tsp black pepper (1g)
- 1/8 tsp salt (0.5g)

Instructions:

1. Preheat oven to 375°F (190°C).
2. Roast seasoned eggplant slices for 10-12 minutes until tender.
3. Meanwhile, scramble the eggs in a pan.
4. Top the roasted eggplant slices with scrambled eggs and sprinkle Parmesan cheese on top.
5. Bake for 3-5 minutes until the cheese is melted.

Nutritional Facts (Per Serving): Calories: 400 | Carbohydrates: 8g | Protein: 21g | Fat: 17g | Sugars: 3g | Fiber: 4g | Sodium: 380mg

Glycemic Index: Eggplant: Low (GI = 15) | Eggs: Negligible GI | Parmesan: Low (GI = 0)

Buckwheat Pancakes with Cinnamon and Walnuts

Prep: 10 minutes | Cook: 10 minutes | Serves: 2

Ingredients:

- 1/2 cup buckwheat flour (60g)
- 2 large eggs (100g)
- 1 tbsp olive oil (15ml)
- 1 tbsp low carb sweetener (5g)
- 1/4 tsp ground cinnamon (1g)
- 1/4 cup chopped walnuts (30g)
- 1/2 tsp baking powder (2g)

Instructions:

1. In a bowl, mix buckwheat flour, eggs, olive oil, low carb sweetener, cinnamon, and baking powder to form a batter.
2. Heat a non-stick pan over medium heat and cook the pancakes for 2-3 minutes on each side until golden brown.
3. Serve the pancakes topped with chopped walnuts.

Nutritional Facts (Per Serving): Calories: 400 | Carbohydrates: 20g | Protein: 18g | Fat: 16g | Sugars: 3g | Fiber: 5g | Sodium: 350mg

Glycemic Index: Buckwheat flour: Low (GI = 49) | Walnuts: Low (GI = 15)

Crustless Quiche with Spinach, Mushrooms, and Feta

Prep: 10 minutes | Cook: 30 minutes | Serves: 2

Ingredients:

- 4 large eggs (200g)
- 1 cup fresh spinach, chopped (30g)
- 1 cup sliced mushrooms (100g)
- 1/4 cup crumbled feta cheese (60g)
- 1 tbsp olive oil (15ml)
- 1/4 tsp black pepper (1g)
- 1/8 tsp salt (0.5g)

Instructions:

1. Preheat oven to 375°F (190°C).
2. Heat olive oil in a pan over medium heat and sauté mushrooms for 5 minutes until softened.
3. In a bowl, whisk eggs, black pepper, and salt. Stir in spinach, sautéed mushrooms, and crumbled feta.
4. Pour the mixture into a greased baking dish and bake for 25-30 minutes until set.
5. Serve warm.

Nutritional Facts (Per Serving): Calories: 400 | Carbohydrates: 6g | Protein: 20g | Fat: 17g | Sugars: 2g | Fiber: 2g | Sodium: 400mg

Glycemic Index: Eggs: Negligible GI | Spinach: Low (GI = 15) | Mushrooms: Low (GI = 15) | Feta: Low (GI = 0)

Baked Zucchini Turkey Fritters

Prep: 10 minutes | Cook: 18 minutes | Serves: 2

Ingredients:

- 3 oz ground turkey (85g)
- 1/2 cup grated zucchini (60g)
- 1 tbsp almond flour (10g)
- 1 large egg (50g)
- 1/2 tbsp olive oil (7ml)
- 1/4 tsp garlic powder (0.5g)
- 1/4 tsp black pepper (1g)
- 1/8 tsp salt (0.5g)

Instructions:

1. Preheat oven to 375°F (190°C).
2. Mix all ingredients in a bowl. Form 2 small fritters.
3. Line a baking tray with parchment, brush with olive oil.
4. Bake fritters for 18 minutes, flipping once halfway.
5. Serve with a spoon of Greek yogurt or fresh herbs.

Nutritional Facts (Per Serving): Calories: 398 | Carbohydrates: 7g | Protein: 24g | Fat: 17g | Sugar: 2g | Fiber: 2g | Sodium: 410mg

Glycemic Index: Turkey: 0 | Zucchini: 15 | Almond flour: 10

Coconut Yogurt Parfait with Berries and Seeds

Prep: 5 minutes | Cook: None | Serves: 1

Ingredients:

- 1/2 cup unsweetened coconut yogurt (120g)
- 1/4 cup mixed berries (blueberries, raspberries – 50g)
- 1 tbsp ground flaxseeds (10g)
- 1 tsp chia seeds (4g)
- 1/2 tsp cinnamon (1g)
- 1 tsp monk fruit sweetener (2g)

Instructions:

1. In a glass or bowl, layer yogurt, berries, and seeds.
2. Sprinkle with cinnamon and monk fruit sweetener.
3. Let sit for 5 minutes before serving.

Nutritional Facts (Per Serving): Calories: 378 | Carbohydrates: 19g | Protein: 10g | Fat: 17g | Sugar: 5g | Fiber: 7g | Sodium: 190mg

Glycemic Index: Coconut yogurt: 35 | Berries: 30–40 | Seeds: 1

Egg-Stuffed Bell Pepper Boats

Prep: 10 minutes | Cook: 20 minutes | Serves: 2

Ingredients:

- 1 medium red bell pepper, halved and seeded (100g)
- 2 large eggs (100g)
- 1 tbsp crumbled feta (15g)
- 1 tsp olive oil (5ml)
- 1/4 tsp oregano (0.5g)
- 1/4 tsp black pepper (1g)
- 1/8 tsp salt (0.5g)

Instructions:

1. Preheat oven to 375°F (190°C).
2. Place pepper halves in a baking dish.
3. Drizzle with olive oil and season with salt, pepper, and oregano.
4. Crack one egg into each half.
5. Sprinkle with feta and bake 18–20 minutes until eggs are set.

Nutritional Facts (Per Serving): Calories: 390 | Carbohydrates: 7g | Protein: 21g | Fat: 17g | Sugar: 3g | Fiber: 2g | Sodium: 420mg

Glycemic Index: Egg: 0 | Bell pepper: 15 | Feta: 0

Mini Broccoli and Cheese Casserole

Prep: 10 minutes | Cook: 20 minutes | Serves: 1

Ingredients:

- 1/2 cup steamed broccoli florets (75g)
- 1/2 cup low-fat cottage cheese (100g)
- 1 large egg (50g)
- 2 tbsp shredded mozzarella (30g)
- 1/4 tsp onion powder (0.5g)
- 1/4 tsp black pepper (1g)
- 1/8 tsp salt (0.5g)

Instructions:

1. Preheat oven to 375°F (190°C).
2. In a bowl, mix all ingredients.
3. Pour into a small baking dish or ramekin.
4. Bake for 20 minutes until golden and set.
5. Serve warm.

Nutritional Facts (Per Serving): Calories: 392 | Carbohydrates: 8g | Protein: 24g | Fat: 17g | Sugar: 3g | Fiber: 2g | Sodium: 430mg

Glycemic Index: Broccoli: 15 | Cottage cheese: 30 | Mozzarella: 0

Warm Chia Almond Porridge with Berries

Prep: 5 minutes | Cook: 5 minutes | Serves: 1

Ingredients:

- 1 cup unsweetened almond milk (240ml)
- 2 tbsp chia seeds (20g)
- 1 tbsp ground almonds (10g)
- 1/4 cup mixed fresh berries (50g)
- 1/2 tsp cinnamon (1.5g)
- 1 tsp monk fruit sweetener (2g)

Instructions:

1. In a saucepan, heat almond milk until warm.
2. Stir in chia seeds, almonds, cinnamon, and sweetener. Simmer for 3–4 minutes.
3. Pour into a bowl, top with berries, and serve.

Nutritional Facts (Per Serving): Calories: 385 | Carbohydrates: 18g | Protein: 10g | Fat: 17g | Sugar: 4g | Fiber: 8g | Sodium: 190mg

Glycemic Index: Chia: 1 | Almond milk: 25 | Berries: 30–40

Eggplant and Goat Cheese Stack

Prep: 10 minutes | Cook: 15 minutes | Serves: 1

Ingredients:

- 4 slices eggplant (120g)
- 1 tbsp goat cheese (15g)
- 1/2 tbsp olive oil (7ml)
- 1/2 tsp balsamic vinegar (2.5ml)
- 1/4 tsp dried basil (0.5g)
- 1/4 tsp black pepper (1g)
- 1/8 tsp salt (0.5g)

Instructions:

1. Brush eggplant slices with olive oil and roast in a skillet or oven for 5–6 minutes per side.
2. Stack slices with a smear of goat cheese between layers.
3. Drizzle with balsamic vinegar and sprinkle herbs.
4. Serve warm as a brunch starter.

Nutritional Facts (Per Serving): Calories: 375 | Carbohydrates: 11g | Protein: 11g | Fat: 17g | Sugar: 4g | Fiber: 4g | Sodium: 300mg

Glycemic Index: Eggplant: 15 | Goat cheese: 0 | Olive oil: 0

Turkey, Arugula & Avocado Lettuce Wraps

Prep: 8 minutes | Cook: 5 minutes | Serves: 2

Ingredients:

- 3 oz cooked turkey breast, sliced (85g)
- 2 large romaine lettuce leaves (30g)
- 1/4 avocado, sliced (50g)
- 1/4 cup arugula (10g)
- 1 tsp Dijon mustard (5g)
- 1/2 tbsp olive oil (7ml)
- 1/4 tsp black pepper (1g)
- 1/8 tsp salt (0.5g)

Instructions:

1. Warm the turkey slices in a pan or microwave (optional).
2. Lay out lettuce leaves. Spread mustard inside.
3. Fill with turkey, avocado, and arugula.
4. Drizzle olive oil, season with salt and pepper.
5. Roll gently and serve.

Nutritional Facts (Per Serving): Calories: 388 | Carbohydrates: 7g | Protein: 23g | Fat: 18g | Sugar: 1g | Fiber: 3g | Sodium: 430mg

Glycemic Index: Turkey: 0 | Lettuce: 15 | Avocado: 15

Stuffed Portobello Mushrooms with Egg

Prep: 10 minutes | Cook: 15 minutes | Serves: 1

Ingredients:

- 2 medium Portobello mushroom caps (100g)
- 2 small eggs (90g)
- 1 tbsp grated Parmesan cheese (7g)
- 1 tsp olive oil (5ml)
- 1/4 tsp black pepper (1g)
- 1/8 tsp salt (0.5g)

Instructions:

1. Preheat oven to 375°F (190°C).
2. Brush mushrooms with olive oil, place on a baking tray.
3. Crack one egg into each cap, season with salt and pepper.
4. Top with grated Parmesan and bake for 15 minutes.
5. Serve warm.

Nutritional Facts (Per Serving): Calories: 392 | Carbohydrates: 5g | Protein: 22g | Fat: 18g | Sugar: 2g | Fiber: 2g | Sodium: 420mg

Glycemic Index: Mushrooms: 10 | Eggs: 0 | Parmesan: 0

CHAPTER 4: LUNCH: Hearty Soups and Stews for Balanced Blood Sugar

Beef and Vegetable Stew with Carrots and Celery

Prep: 20 minutes | Cook: 40 minutes | Serves: 2

Ingredients:

- 8 oz beef sirloin (225g)
- 1 medium carrot, sliced (100g)
- 2 stalks celery, chopped (80g)
- 1 cup beef broth, low sodium (240ml)
- 1 tbsp olive oil (15ml)
- 1 small onion, diced (70g)
- 2 cloves garlic, minced (5g)
- 1 tsp dried thyme (2g)
- Salt and pepper to taste

Instructions:

1. Brown beef in oil (5–7 min).
2. Add onion & garlic, sauté 3 min.
3. Add carrots, celery, thyme. Cook 5 min.
4. Add broth, simmer 25–30 min.
5. Season & serve.

Nutritional Facts (Per Serving): Calories: 500 | Carbohydrates: 15g | Protein: 23g | Fat: 20g | Fiber: 4g | Sugar: 5g | Sodium: 600mg

Glycemic Index: Carrot: Medium (GI = 47) | Celery: Low (GI = 15)

Creamy Cauliflower and Leek Soup with Roasted Garlic

Prep: 15 minutes | Cook: 30 minutes | Serves: 2

Ingredients:

- 2 cups cauliflower florets (300g)
- 1 leek, sliced (150g)
- 4 cloves garlic, roasted (10g)
- 1 cup vegetable broth, low sodium (240ml)
- 1/2 cup unsweetened almond milk (120ml)
- 1 tbsp olive oil (15ml)
- 1 tbsp low carb sweetener (optional)
- Salt and pepper to taste

Instructions:

1. Sauté leek in oil (5 min).
2. Add cauliflower & garlic, cook 3 min.
3. Add broth, simmer 20 min.
4. Blend smooth. Stir in almond milk, season.

Nutritional Facts (Per Serving): Calories: 500 | Carbohydrates: 20g | Protein: 22g | Fat: 17g | Fiber: 7g | Sugar: 4g | Sodium: 550mg

Glycemic Index: Cauliflower: Low (GI = 15) | Leek: Low (GI = 15)

Creamy Broccoli and Cauliflower Soup with Almonds

Prep: 15 minutes | Cook: 30 minutes | Serves: 2

Ingredients:

- 1 cup broccoli florets (150g)
- 1 cup cauliflower florets (150g)
- 2 tbsp ground almonds (30g)
- 1 cup vegetable broth, low sodium (240ml)
- 1/2 cup unsweetened almond milk (120ml)
- 1 tbsp olive oil (15ml)
- 2 cloves garlic, minced (5g)
- 1 tsp dried basil (2g)
- Salt and pepper to taste

Instructions:

1. Heat olive oil in a pot over medium heat. Add garlic and cook until fragrant, about 1 minute.
2. Add broccoli, cauliflower, and basil, cook for 5 minutes.
3. Pour in vegetable broth, bring to a boil, then reduce heat and simmer for 20 minutes until vegetables are tender.
4. Blend the soup until smooth. Stir in almond milk and ground almonds. Season with salt and pepper.

Nutritional Facts (Per Serving): Calories: 500 | Carbohydrates: 18g | Protein: 21g | Fat: 20g | Fiber: 6g | Sugar: 4g | Sodium: 550mg

Glycemic Index: Broccoli: Low (GI = 15) | Cauliflower: Low (GI = 15) | Almonds: Low (GI = 0)

Chicken and Quinoa Soup with Spinach and Herbs

Prep: 15 minutes | Cook: 25 minutes | Serves: 2

Ingredients:

- 6 oz chicken breast, diced (170g)
- 1/4 cup quinoa (45g)
- 1 cup spinach, chopped (30g)
- 4 cups low sodium chicken broth (960ml)
- 1 small onion, diced (70g)
- 1 tbsp olive oil (15ml)
- 2 cloves garlic, minced (5g)
- 1 tsp dried oregano (2g)
- 1 tbsp fresh parsley, chopped (15g)
- Salt and pepper to taste

Instructions:

1. Heat olive oil in a pot over medium heat. Add chicken and cook until browned, about 5-7 minutes.
2. Add onion and garlic, cook until softened, about 3 minutes.
3. Stir in quinoa, chicken broth, oregano, and parsley. Bring to a boil, then simmer for 15 minutes.
4. Add spinach and cook for another 2-3 minutes until wilted. Season with salt and pepper.

Nutritional Facts (Per Serving): Calories: 500 | Carbohydrates: 22g | Protein: 24g | Fat: 18g | Fiber: 4g | Sugar: 3g | Sodium: 650mg

Glycemic Index: Quinoa: Low (GI = 53) | Spinach: Low (GI = 15)

Chicken and Lentil Stew

Prep: 20 minutes | Cook: 35 minutes | Serves: 2

Ingredients:

- 6 oz chicken thighs, diced (170g)
- 1/2 cup red lentils (100g)
- 1 small carrot, diced (100g)
- 1 stalk celery, chopped (40g)
- 1 small onion, diced (70g)
- 2 cups low sodium chicken broth (480ml)
- 1 tbsp olive oil (15ml)
- 1 tsp ground cumin (2g)
- 1 tsp paprika (2g)
- Salt and pepper to taste

Instructions:

1. Heat olive oil in a pot over medium heat. Add chicken and cook until browned, about 5-7 minutes.
2. Add onion, carrot, and celery, cook until softened, about 5 minutes.
3. Stir in lentils, cumin, and paprika. Add chicken broth, bring to a boil, then reduce heat and simmer for 25 minutes until lentils are tender.
4. Season with salt and pepper before serving.

Nutritional Facts (Per Serving): Calories: 500 | Carbohydrates: 28g | Protein: 23g | Fat: 18g | Fiber: 6g | Sugar: 4g | Sodium: 600mg

Glycemic Index: Lentils: Low (GI = 32) | Carrot: Medium (GI = 47)

Butternut Squash and Turkey Chili

Prep: 20 minutes | Cook: 40 minutes | Serves: 2

Ingredients:

- 6 oz ground turkey (170g)
- 1 cup butternut squash, diced (150g)
- 1/2 cup canned diced tomatoes, no salt added (120g)
- 1 small bell pepper, chopped (100g)
- 1 cup low sodium chicken broth (240ml)
- 1 tbsp olive oil (15ml)
- 1 tsp chili powder (2g)
- 1/2 tsp ground cumin (1g)
- 1 clove garlic, minced (2g)
- Salt and pepper to taste

Instructions:

1. Heat olive oil in a pot over medium heat.
2. Add ground turkey and cook until browned, about 5-7 minutes.
3. Add garlic and bell pepper, cook until softened, about 3 minutes.
4. Stir in butternut squash, tomatoes, chili powder, cumin, and chicken broth. Bring to a boil, then reduce heat and simmer for 25-30 minutes until squash is tender.
5. Season with salt and pepper.

Nutritional Facts (Per Serving): Calories: 500 | Carbohydrates: 25g | Protein: 24g | Fat: 19g | Fiber: 7g | Sugar: 5g | Sodium: 550mg

Glycemic Index: Butternut Squash: Medium (GI = 51) | Bell Pepper: Low (GI = 15)

Beef and Barley Soup with Root Vegetables

Prep: 15 minutes | Cook: 40 minutes | Serves: 2

Ingredients:

- 6 oz lean beef chuck, diced (170g)
- 1/4 cup pearl barley (50g)
- 1 small carrot, diced (100g)
- 1 small parsnip, diced (100g)
- 1 small onion, diced (70g)
- 3 cups low sodium beef broth (720ml)
- 1 tbsp olive oil (15ml)
- 1 tsp dried thyme (2g)
- Salt and pepper to taste

Instructions:

1. Heat olive oil in a pot over medium heat. Add beef and cook until browned, about 5-7 minutes.
2. Add onion, carrot, and parsnip, sauté for 5 minutes until softened.
3. Stir in barley, thyme, and beef broth. Bring to a boil, then reduce heat and simmer for 30 minutes until barley is tender and beef is cooked through.
4. Season with salt and pepper to taste.

Nutritional Facts (Per Serving): Calories: 500 | Carbohydrates: 28g | Protein: 24g | Fat: 18g | Fiber: 6g | Sugar: 4g | Sodium: 600mg

Glycemic Index: Barley: Low (GI = 28) | Carrot: Medium (GI = 47) | Parsnip: Medium (GI = 52)

Turkey and White Bean Soup with Fresh Cilantro

Prep: 10 minutes | Cook: 30 minutes | Serves: 2

Ingredients:

- 6 oz ground turkey (170g)
- 1/2 cup canned white beans, rinsed (120g)
- 1 small onion, diced (70g)
- 1 small bell pepper, diced (100g)
- 2 cloves garlic, minced (5g)
- 3 cups low sodium chicken broth (720ml)
- 1 tbsp olive oil (15ml)
- 1 tsp ground cumin (2g)
- 2 tbsp fresh cilantro, chopped (15g)
- Salt and pepper to taste

Instructions:

1. Heat olive oil in a pot over medium heat. Add ground turkey and cook until browned, about 5-7 minutes.
2. Add onion, bell pepper, and garlic, sauté for 5 minutes.
3. Stir in white beans, cumin, and chicken broth. Bring to a boil, then reduce heat and simmer for 20 minutes.
4. Garnish with fresh cilantro and season with salt and pepper before serving.

Nutritional Facts (Per Serving): Calories: 500 | Carbohydrates: 24g | Protein: 23g | Fat: 19g | Fiber: 7g | Sugar: 3g | Sodium: 550mg

Glycemic Index: White Beans: Low (GI = 31) | Bell Pepper: Low (GI = 15)

Vegetable and Ground Beef Stew with Zucchini

Prep: 15 minutes | Cook: 35 minutes | Serves: 2

Ingredients:

- 6 oz lean ground beef (170g)
- 1 small zucchini, chopped (150g)
- 1 small carrot, diced (100g)
- 1 small bell pepper, diced (100g)
- 1 small onion, diced (70g)
- 2 cups low sodium beef broth (480ml)
- 1 tbsp olive oil (15ml)
- 1 tsp paprika (2g)
- Salt and pepper to taste

Instructions:

1. Heat olive oil in a pot over medium heat. Add ground beef and cook until browned, about 5-7 minutes.
2. Add onion, carrot, bell pepper, and zucchini, sauté for 5 minutes.
3. Stir in paprika and beef broth. Bring to a boil, then reduce heat and simmer for 25-30 minutes until vegetables are tender.
4. Season with salt and pepper before serving.

Nutritional Facts (Per Serving): Calories: 500 | Carbohydrates: 20g | Protein: 24g | Fat: 20g | Fiber: 5g | Sugar: 4g | Sodium: 600mg

Glycemic Index: Zucchini: Low (GI = 15) | Carrot: Medium (GI = 47)

Savory Beef and Mushroom Stew with Fresh Thyme

Prep: 15 minutes | Cook: 40 minutes | Serves: 2

Ingredients:

- 6 oz lean beef chuck, diced (170g)
- 1 cup mushrooms, sliced (150g)
- 1 small onion, diced (70g)
- 2 cloves garlic, minced (5g)
- 3 cups low sodium beef broth (720ml)
- 1 tbsp olive oil (15ml)
- 1 tsp fresh thyme (2g)
- Salt and pepper to taste

Instructions:

1. Heat olive oil in a pot over medium heat. Add beef and cook until browned, about 5-7 minutes.
2. Add onion and garlic, cook until softened, about 3 minutes.
3. Stir in mushrooms and thyme, cook for another 5 minutes.
4. Pour in beef broth, bring to a boil, then reduce heat and simmer for 30 minutes until beef is tender.
5. Season with salt and pepper before serving.

Nutritional Facts (Per Serving): Calories: 500 | Carbohydrates: 15g | Protein: 23g | Fat: 20g | Fiber: 3g | Sugar: 4g | Sodium: 600mg

Glycemic Index: Mushrooms: Low (GI = 15) | Onion: Low (GI = 10)

Root Vegetable and Beef Stew with Fresh Parsley

Prep: 20 minutes | Cook: 45 minutes | Serves: 2

Ingredients:

- 6 oz lean beef stew meat, diced (170g)
- 1 small carrot, diced (100g)
- 1 small parsnip, diced (100g)
- 1 small turnip, diced (100g)
- 1 small onion, diced (70g)
- 3 cups low sodium beef broth (720ml)
- 1 tbsp olive oil (15ml)
- 2 tbsp fresh parsley, chopped (15g)
- Salt and pepper to taste

Instructions:

1. Heat olive oil in a pot over medium heat. Add beef and cook until browned, about 5-7 minutes.
2. Add onion, carrot, parsnip, and turnip, sauté for 5 minutes until softened.
3. Stir in beef broth, bring to a boil, then reduce heat and simmer for 35 minutes until vegetables are tender.
4. Stir in fresh parsley and season with salt and pepper before serving.

Nutritional Facts (Per Serving): Calories: 500 | Carbohydrates: 28g | Protein: 23g | Fat: 19g | Fiber: 6g | Sugar: 5g | Sodium: 650mg

Glycemic Index: Carrot: Medium (GI = 47) | Parsnip: Medium (GI = 52) | Turnip: Low (GI = 30)

Creamy Mushroom Soup with Roasted Garlic and Herbs

Prep: 15 minutes | Cook: 30 minutes | Serves: 2

Ingredients:

- 1 cup mushrooms, sliced (150g)
- 1 small leek, sliced (150g)
- 4 cloves garlic, roasted (10g)
- 2 cups low sodium vegetable broth (480ml)
- 1/2 cup unsweetened almond milk (120ml)
- 1 tbsp olive oil (15ml)
- 1 tsp fresh thyme (2g)
- Salt and pepper to taste

Instructions:

1. Heat olive oil in a pot over medium heat. Add leek and mushrooms, cook until softened, about 5 minutes.
2. Stir in roasted garlic and thyme, cook for another 2 minutes.
3. Pour in vegetable broth, bring to a boil, then reduce heat and simmer for 20 minutes.
4. Blend the soup until smooth, then stir in almond milk. Season with salt and pepper before serving.

Nutritional Facts (Per Serving): Calories: 500 | Carbohydrates: 20g | Protein: 22g | Fat: 19g | Fiber: 4g | Sugar: 3g | Sodium: 550mg

Glycemic Index: Mushrooms: Low (GI = 15) | Leek: Low (GI = 15)

Tomato and Red Lentil Soup with Fresh Basil

Prep: 10 minutes | Cook: 20 minutes | Serves: 1

Ingredients:

- 1/4 cup red lentils (50g)
- 1/2 cup canned diced tomatoes, no salt (120g)
- 1/2 small onion, chopped (35g)
- 1 tsp olive oil (5ml)
- 1 cup low sodium vegetable broth (240ml)
- 1 clove garlic, minced (2g)
- 1 tbsp fresh basil, chopped (5g)
- 1/4 tsp black pepper (1g)
- 1/8 tsp salt (0.5g)

Instructions:

1. In a pot, heat olive oil and sauté onion and garlic for 3 minutes.
2. Add lentils, tomatoes, and broth. Bring to a boil.
3. Reduce heat and simmer for 15 minutes until lentils are tender.
4. Stir in basil, season with salt and pepper, and serve.

Nutritional Facts (Per Serving): Calories: 398 | Carbohydrates: 28g | Protein: 21g | Fat: 14g | Sugar: 4g | Fiber: 6g | Sodium: 440mg

Glycemic Index: Lentils: 32 | Tomatoes: 30 | Onion: 10

Green Vegetable Stew with Chicken and Dill

Prep: 10 minutes | Cook: 20 minutes | Serves: 1

Ingredients:

- 4 oz chicken breast, diced (115g)
- 1/2 cup chopped green beans (60g)
- 1/2 cup chopped zucchini (60g)
- 1/2 cup spinach (15g)
- 1 1/2 cups low sodium chicken broth (360ml)
- 1 tsp olive oil (5ml)
- 1 tbsp fresh dill, chopped (5g)
- 1/4 tsp garlic powder (0.5g)
- 1/4 tsp black pepper (1g)
- 1/8 tsp salt (0.5g)

Instructions:

1. Heat olive oil in a pot. Add chicken, cook 5 minutes.
2. Add green beans and zucchini. Sauté for 3–4 minutes.
3. Add broth and garlic powder. Simmer for 10 minutes.
4. Stir in spinach and dill. Cook 1 minute. Season and serve.

Nutritional Facts (Per Serving): Calories: 392 | Carbohydrates: 9g | Protein: 24g | Fat: 17g | Sugar: 3g | Fiber: 3g | Sodium: 420mg

Glycemic Index: Chicken: 0 | Green beans: 15 | Zucchini: 15 | Spinach: 15

Egg Drop Soup with Mushrooms and Bok Choy

Prep: 5 minutes | Cook: 10 minutes | Serves: 1

Ingredients:

- 1 large egg, beaten (50g)
- 1/2 cup sliced mushrooms (50g)
- 1/2 cup chopped bok choy (50g)
- 1 1/2 cups low sodium vegetable broth (360ml)
- 1/2 tsp sesame oil (2ml)
- 1 tsp soy sauce, low sodium (5ml)
- 1/4 tsp ground ginger (0.5g)
- 1/8 tsp salt (0.5g)
- 1/4 tsp white pepper (1g)

Instructions:

1. Bring broth to a simmer in a saucepan. Add mushrooms, bok choy, ginger, soy sauce, salt and pepper. Cook 5 minutes.
2. Slowly drizzle in beaten egg while stirring broth in a circular motion.
3. Cook 1 more minute. Stir in sesame oil. Serve hot.

Nutritional Facts (Per Serving): Calories: 380 | Carbohydrates: 7g | Protein: 20g | Fat: 17g | Sugar: 2g | Fiber: 2g | Sodium: 430mg

Glycemic Index: Egg: 0 | Mushrooms: 15 | Bok choy: 15

Turkey and Spinach Soup with Lemon

Prep: 10 minutes | **Cook:** 15 minutes | **Serves:** 1

Ingredients:

- 4 oz ground turkey (115g)
- 1/2 cup chopped spinach (30g)
- 1/4 cup diced carrots (30g)
- 1 1/2 cups low sodium chicken broth (360ml)
- 1 tbsp lemon juice (15ml)
- 1 tsp olive oil (5ml)
- 1/4 tsp dried oregano (0.5g)
- 1/4 tsp black pepper (1g)
- 1/8 tsp salt (0.5g)

Instructions:

1. Heat olive oil in a pot. Add turkey and cook 5 minutes.

2. Add carrots and broth. Simmer for 8–10 minutes.
3. Stir in spinach, oregano, lemon juice, and seasonings. Cook 1 more minute and serve.

Nutritional Facts (Per Serving): Calories: 390 | Carbohydrates: 9g | Protein: 24g | Fat: 17g | Sugar: 3g | Fiber: 2g | Sodium: 430mg

Glycemic Index: Turkey: 0 | Carrot: 47 | Spinach: 15

Cabbage and Beef Tomato Stew

Prep: 10 minutes | **Cook:** 20 minutes | **Serves:** 1

Ingredients:

- 4 oz lean ground beef (115g)
- 1 cup shredded white cabbage (70g)
- 1/2 cup canned diced tomatoes, no salt (120g)
- 1/2 small onion, chopped (35g)
- 1 tsp olive oil (5ml)
- 1/4 tsp smoked paprika (0.5g)
- 1/4 tsp black pepper (1g)
- 1/8 tsp salt (0.5g)

Instructions:

1. In a pot, sauté onion and beef in olive oil for 5–6 minutes.
2. Add cabbage, tomatoes, and spices. Cook on low heat for 10–12 minutes, stirring occasionally.
3. Serve hot.

Nutritional Facts (Per Serving): Calories: 395 | Carbohydrates: 10g | Protein: 23g | Fat: 18g | Sugar: 4g | Fiber: 3g | Sodium: 440mg

Glycemic Index: Beef: 0 | Cabbage: 15 | Tomato: 30

Creamy Turnip and Leek Soup

Prep: 10 minutes | **Cook:** 20 minutes | **Serves:** 1

Ingredients:

- 1/2 cup diced turnip (70g)
- 1/2 cup sliced leeks (75g)
- 1/2 tbsp olive oil (7ml)
- 1 cup low sodium vegetable broth (240ml)
- 1/4 cup unsweetened almond milk (60ml)
- 1/2 clove garlic, minced (2g)
- 1/4 tsp dried thyme (0.5g)
- 1/4 tsp black pepper (1g)
- 1/8 tsp salt (0.5g)

Instructions:

1. Sauté leeks and garlic in olive oil for 3–4 minutes.
2. Add turnip, broth, thyme, salt and pepper. Simmer 12–15 minutes.
3. Blend until smooth, stir in almond milk, and reheat gently. Serve warm.

Nutritional Facts (Per Serving): Calories: 382 | Carbohydrates: 14g | Protein: 20g | Fat: 17g | Sugar: 3g | Fiber: 4g | Sodium: 420mg

Glycemic Index: Turnip: 30 | Leek: 15 | Almond milk: 25

Eggplant Chickpea Stew with Tahini

Prep: 10 minutes | Cook: 20 minutes | Serves: 1

Ingredients:

- 1/2 cup diced eggplant (75g)
- 1/4 cup canned chickpeas, rinsed (60g)
- 1/4 cup canned diced tomatoes (60g)
- 1/2 small onion, chopped (35g)
- 1 tsp olive oil (5ml)
- 1 tsp tahini (5g)
- 1/4 tsp cumin (0.5g)
- 1/4 tsp black pepper (1g)
- 1/8 tsp salt (0.5g)
- 1/2 cup low sodium vegetable broth (120ml)

Instructions:

1. Heat olive oil in a saucepan. Sauté onion and eggplant 5 minutes.
2. Add tomatoes, chickpeas, broth, cumin, salt, and pepper. Simmer for 10–12 minutes.
3. Stir in tahini before serving.

Nutritional Facts (Per Serving): Calories: 388 | Carbohydrates: 21g | Protein: 18g | Fat: 17g | Sugar: 4g | Fiber: 5g | Sodium: 430mg

Glycemic Index: Chickpeas: 28 | Eggplant: 15 | Tahini: 35

Garlic Turkey Meatball Soup with Greens

Prep: 12 minutes | Cook: 15 minutes | Serves: 1

Ingredients:

- 3 oz ground turkey (85g)
- 1 tbsp almond flour (10g)
- 1 clove garlic, minced (3g)
- 1 cup spinach (30g)
- 1 1/2 cups low sodium chicken broth (360ml)
- 1/4 tsp oregano (0.5g)
- 1/2 tbsp olive oil (7ml)
- 1/4 tsp black pepper (1g)
- 1/8 tsp salt (0.5g)

Instructions:

1. Mix turkey, almond flour, garlic, salt and pepper. Form small meatballs.
2. Heat olive oil in a pot, brown meatballs 4–5 minutes.
3. Add broth and oregano, simmer 10 minutes.
4. Stir in spinach for final 1–2 minutes. Serve hot.

Nutritional Facts (Per Serving): Calories: 395 | Carbohydrates: 7g | Protein: 24g | Fat: 18g | Sugar: 2g | Fiber: 2g | Sodium: 430mg

Glycemic Index: Turkey: 0 | Almond flour: 10 | Spinach: 15

Zucchini and Herb Soup with Poached Egg

Prep: 7 minutes | Cook: 15 minutes | Serves: 1

Ingredients:

- 1/2 cup sliced zucchini (60g)
- 1 cup low sodium vegetable broth (240ml)
- 1 egg (50g)
- 1 tbsp fresh parsley, chopped (5g)
- 1/2 tsp olive oil (2ml)
- 1/4 tsp garlic powder (0.5g)
- 1/4 tsp black pepper (1g)
- 1/8 tsp salt (0.5g)

Instructions:

1. In a saucepan, bring broth to a simmer. Add zucchini, garlic powder, and cook 5 minutes.
2. Poach egg directly in broth for 4–5 minutes until set.
3. Stir in parsley, season with salt and pepper, drizzle olive oil, and serve.

Nutritional Facts (Per Serving): Calories: 379 | Carbohydrates: 6g | Protein: 21g | Fat: 17g | Sugar: 2g | Fiber: 2g | Sodium: 400mg

Glycemic Index: Egg: 0 | Zucchini: 15 | Parsley: 15

Low-Glycemic Grain Bowls

Bulgur Wheat Bowl with Ground Turkey and Zucchini

Prep: 15 minutes | **Cook:** 20 minutes | **Serves:** 2

Ingredients:

- 1/2 cup bulgur wheat (90g)
- 6 oz ground turkey (170g)
- 1 small zucchini, chopped (150g)
- 1 small onion, diced (70g)
- 1 tbsp olive oil (15ml)
- 1 tsp ground cumin (2g)
- Salt and pepper to taste

Instructions:

1. Cook bulgur wheat according to package instructions.
2. Heat olive oil in a pan over medium heat. Add ground turkey, cook until browned, about 5-7 minutes.
3. Add onion and zucchini, sauté for 5 minutes until softened.
4. Stir in cumin and season with salt and pepper.
5. Serve the turkey mixture over cooked bulgur wheat.

Nutritional Facts (Per Serving): Calories: 500 | Carbohydrates: 27g | Protein: 24g | Fat: 19g | Fiber: 7g | Sugar: 3g | Sodium: 600mg

Glycemic Index: Bulgur: Low (GI = 48) | Zucchini: Low (GI = 15)

Millet and Carrot Bowl with Turkey Meatballs

Prep: 20 minutes | **Cook:** 30 minutes | **Serves:** 2

Ingredients:

- 1/2 cup millet (100g)
- 6 oz ground turkey (170g)
- 1 small carrot, grated (100g)
- 1 small onion, diced (70g)
- 1 egg (50g)
- 1 tbsp olive oil (15ml)
- 1 tsp paprika (2g)
- Salt and pepper to taste

Instructions:

1. Cook millet according to package instructions.
2. In a bowl, mix ground turkey, grated carrot, onion, egg, paprika, salt, and pepper. Form into small meatballs.
3. Heat olive oil in a pan over medium heat and cook the meatballs for 8-10 minutes, turning occasionally until browned and cooked through.
4. Serve the turkey meatballs over cooked millet.

Nutritional Facts (Per Serving): Calories: 500 | Carbohydrates: 25g | Protein: 23g | Fat: 19g | Fiber: 5g | Sugar: 3g | Sodium: 550mg

Glycemic Index: Millet: Medium (GI = 71) | Carrot: Medium (GI = 47)

Farro and Grilled Vegetables with a Yogurt-Tahini Dressing

Prep: 20 minutes | **Cook:** 25 minutes | **Serves:** 2

Ingredients:

- 1/2 cup farro (100g)
- 1 small eggplant, chopped (150g)
- 1 small zucchini, chopped (150g)
- 1 small bell pepper, chopped (100g)
- 1 tbsp olive oil (15ml)
- 2 tbsp plain Greek yogurt (30g)
- 1 tbsp tahini (15g)
- 1 tbsp lemon juice (15ml)
- Salt and pepper to taste

Instructions:

1. Cook farro according to package instructions.
2. Toss eggplant, zucchini, and bell pepper with olive oil, salt, and pepper. Grill the vegetables until tender, about 5-7 minutes per side.
3. In a small bowl, whisk together yogurt, tahini, lemon juice, salt, and pepper for the dressing.
4. Serve the grilled vegetables over farro and drizzle with yogurt-tahini dressing.

Nutritional Facts (Per Serving): Calories: 500 | Carbohydrates: 30g | Protein: 22g | Fat: 19g | Fiber: 7g | Sugar: 5g | Sodium: 550mg

Glycemic Index: Farro: Medium (GI = 45) | Zucchini: Low (GI = 15) | Bell Pepper: Low (GI = 15)

Quinoa Bowl with Grilled Chicken and Roasted Peppers

Prep: 15 minutes | Cook: 25 minutes | Serves: 2

Ingredients:

- 1/2 cup quinoa (90g)
- 6 oz grilled chicken breast, sliced (170g)
- 1 small red bell pepper, roasted (100g)
- 1 small yellow bell pepper, roasted (100g)
- 1 tbsp olive oil (15ml)
- 1 tsp dried oregano (2g)
- Salt and pepper to taste

Instructions:

1. Cook quinoa according to package instructions.
2. Toss bell peppers with olive oil, oregano, salt, and pepper. Roast in a preheated oven at 400°F (200°C) for 20 minutes, turning halfway through.
3. Grill chicken over medium heat until fully cooked, about 6-8 minutes per side.
4. Serve the quinoa topped with sliced grilled chicken and roasted peppers.

Nutritional Facts (Per Serving): Calories: 500 | Carbohydrates: 24g | Protein: 23g | Fat: 19g | Fiber: 6g | Sugar: 5g | Sodium: 600mg

Glycemic Index: Quinoa: Low (GI = 53) | Bell Pepper: Low (GI = 15)

Barley and Mushroom Bowl with Baby Kale

Prep: 15 minutes | Cook: 30 minutes | Serves: 2

Ingredients:

- 1/2 cup pearl barley (100g)
- 1 cup mushrooms, sliced (150g)
- 2 cups baby kale (60g)
- 1 small onion, diced (70g)
- 1 tbsp olive oil (15ml)
- 1 tsp garlic powder (2g)
- Salt and pepper to taste

Instructions:

1. Cook barley according to package instructions.
2. Heat olive oil in a pan over medium heat. Add onions and mushrooms, sauté for 5-7 minutes until softened.
3. Stir in garlic powder and baby kale, cooking until the kale wilts, about 2 minutes.
4. Serve the sautéed vegetables over cooked barley.

Nutritional Facts (Per Serving): Calories: 500 | Carbohydrates: 28g | Protein: 21g | Fat: 18g | Fiber: 7g | Sugar: 4g | Sodium: 550mg

Glycemic Index: Barley: Low (GI = 28) | Mushrooms: Low (GI = 15) | Kale: Low (GI = 15)

Buckwheat and Roasted Broccoli Bowl with Sunflower Seeds

Prep: 15 minutes | Cook: 25 minutes | Serves: 2

Ingredients:

- 1/2 cup buckwheat groats (100g)
- 1 cup broccoli florets (150g)
- 1 tbsp sunflower seeds (15g)
- 1 small onion, diced (70g)
- 1 tbsp olive oil (15ml)
- 1 tsp lemon juice (5ml)
- Salt and pepper to taste

Instructions:

1. Cook buckwheat according to package instructions.
2. Toss broccoli florets with olive oil, salt, and pepper. Roast in a preheated oven at 400°F (200°C) for 20 minutes.
3. In a pan, toast sunflower seeds until lightly browned, about 2-3 minutes.
4. Serve the roasted broccoli and sunflower seeds over cooked buckwheat, and drizzle with lemon juice.

Nutritional Facts (Per Serving): Calories: 500 | Carbohydrates: 26g | Protein: 22g | Fat: 18g | Fiber: 8g | Sugar: 3g | Sodium: 550mg

Glycemic Index: Buckwheat: Low (GI = 49) | Broccoli: Low (GI = 15) | Sunflower Seeds: Low (GI = 0)

Quinoa and Roasted Veggie Bowl with Tahini Dressing

Prep: 15 minutes | Cook: 25 minutes | Serves: 2

Ingredients:

- 1/2 cup quinoa (90g)
- 1 small zucchini, chopped (150g)
- 1 small red bell pepper, chopped (100g)
- 1 small eggplant, chopped (150g)
- 1 tbsp olive oil (15ml)
- 1 tbsp tahini (15g)
- 1 tbsp lemon juice (15ml)
- 1 tsp low carb sweetener
- Salt and pepper to taste

Instructions:

1. Cook quinoa according to package instructions.
2. Toss zucchini, bell pepper, and eggplant with olive oil, salt, and pepper. Roast in a preheated oven at 400°F (200°C) for 20 minutes.
3. In a small bowl, whisk together tahini, lemon juice, low carb sweetener, salt, and pepper to make the dressing.
4. Serve the quinoa topped with roasted vegetables and drizzle with tahini dressing.

Nutritional Facts (Per Serving): Calories: 500 | Carbohydrates: 27g | Protein: 22g | Fat: 19g | Fiber: 7g | Sugar: 4g | Sodium: 600mg

Glycemic Index: Quinoa: Low (GI = 53) | Zucchini: Low (GI = 15) | Bell Pepper: Low (GI = 15)

Buckwheat Bowl with Grilled Chicken and Avocado

Prep: 15 minutes | Cook: 20 minutes | Serves: 2

Ingredients:

- 1/2 cup buckwheat groats (100g)
- 6 oz grilled chicken breast, sliced (170g)
- 1/2 avocado, sliced (75g)
- 1 small cucumber, sliced (100g)
- 1 tbsp olive oil (15ml)
- 1 tsp lemon juice (5ml)
- Salt and pepper to taste

Instructions:

1. Cook buckwheat according to package instructions.
2. Grill chicken over medium heat until cooked through, about 6-8 minutes per side.
3. Toss cucumber with olive oil, lemon juice, salt, and pepper.
4. Serve the buckwheat topped with grilled chicken, avocado slices, and dressed cucumber.

Nutritional Facts (Per Serving): Calories: 500 | Carbohydrates: 24g | Protein: 24g | Fat: 19g | Fiber: 6g | Sugar: 3g | Sodium: 550mg

Glycemic Index: Buckwheat: Low (GI = 49) | Avocado: Low (GI = 15) | Cucumber: Low (GI = 15)

Millet and Roasted Cauliflower Bowl with Lemon Vinaigrette

Prep: 15 minutes | Cook: 25 minutes | Serves: 2

Ingredients:

- 1/2 cup millet (100g)
- 1 cup cauliflower florets, roasted (150g)
- 1 small onion, diced (70g)
- 1 tbsp sunflower seeds (15g)
- 1 tbsp olive oil (15ml)
- 1 tbsp lemon juice (15ml)
- 1 tsp Dijon mustard (5g)
- Salt and pepper to taste

Instructions:

1. Cook millet according to package instructions.
2. Toss cauliflower with olive oil, salt, and pepper. Roast in a preheated oven at 400°F (200°C) for 20 minutes.
3. In a small bowl, whisk together lemon juice, Dijon mustard, salt, and pepper to make the vinaigrette.
4. Serve the millet topped with roasted cauliflower and sunflower seeds, and drizzle with lemon vinaigrette.

Nutritional Facts (Per Serving): Calories: 500 | Carbohydrates: 28g | Protein: 22g | Fat: 19g | Fiber: 6g | Sugar: 3g | Sodium: 550mg

Glycemic Index: Millet: Medium (GI = 71) | Cauliflower: Low (GI = 15)

Barley and Roasted Red Pepper Bowl with Turkey

Prep: 15 minutes | Cook: 25 minutes | Serves: 2

Ingredients:

- 1/2 cup pearl barley (100g)
- 6 oz ground turkey (170g)
- 1 small red bell pepper, roasted (100g)
- 1 small onion, diced (70g)
- 1 tbsp olive oil (15ml)
- 1 tsp ground cumin (2g)
- Salt and pepper to taste

Instructions:

1. Cook barley according to package instructions.
2. Heat olive oil in a pan over medium heat. Add ground turkey and cook until browned, about 5-7 minutes.
3. Add diced onion and cumin, sauté for 5 minutes until onion is softened.
4. Stir in roasted red pepper and season with salt and pepper.
5. Serve the turkey mixture over cooked barley.

Nutritional Facts (Per Serving): Calories: 500 | Carbohydrates: 26g | Protein: 24g | Fat: 19g | Fiber: 6g | Sugar: 3g | Sodium: 600mg

Glycemic Index: Barley: Low (GI = 28) | Red Bell Pepper: Low (GI = 15)

Quinoa with Sautéed Spinach and Avocado

Prep: 10 minutes | Cook: 15 minutes | Serves: 2

Ingredients:

- 1/2 cup quinoa (90g)
- 1 cup spinach, fresh (30g)
- 1/2 avocado, sliced (75g)
- 1 clove garlic, minced (3g)
- 1 tbsp olive oil (15ml)
- 1 tbsp lemon juice (15ml)
- Salt and pepper to taste

Instructions:

1. Cook quinoa according to package instructions.
2. Heat olive oil in a pan over medium heat. Add garlic and sauté for 1 minute, then add spinach and cook until wilted, about 2 minutes.
3. Serve the quinoa topped with sautéed spinach, avocado slices, and a drizzle of lemon juice. Season with salt and pepper.

Nutritional Facts (Per Serving): Calories: 500 | Carbohydrates: 25g | Protein: 23g | Fat: 19g | Fiber: 7g | Sugar: 2g | Sodium: 550mg

Glycemic Index: Quinoa: Low (GI = 53) | Spinach: Low (GI = 15) | Avocado: Low (GI = 15)

Farro Bowl with Roasted Butternut Squash and Chicken

Prep: 15 minutes | Cook: 25 minutes | Serves: 2

Ingredients:

- 1/2 cup farro (100g)
- 6 oz chicken breast, grilled and sliced (170g)
- 1 cup butternut squash, diced and roasted (150g)
- 1 small onion, diced (70g)
- 1 tbsp olive oil (15ml)
- 1 tsp dried thyme (2g)
- Salt and pepper to taste

Instructions:

1. Cook farro according to package instructions.
2. Toss butternut squash with olive oil, thyme, salt, and pepper. Roast in a preheated oven at 400°F (200°C) for 20 minutes.
3. Grill chicken breast over medium heat until fully cooked, about 6-8 minutes per side.
4. Serve the farro topped with sliced grilled chicken and roasted butternut squash.

Nutritional Facts (Per Serving): Calories: 500 | Carbohydrates: 29g | Protein: 24g | Fat: 18g | Fiber: 6g | Sugar: 3g | Sodium: 550mg

Glycemic Index: Farro: Medium (GI = 45) | Butternut Squash: Medium (GI = 51)

Freekeh Bowl with Roasted Brussels Sprouts and Tahini Drizzle

Prep: 15 minutes | Cook: 20 minutes | Serves: 1

Ingredients:

- 1/4 cup freekeh, uncooked (45g)
- 1 cup Brussels sprouts, halved (120g)
- 1 tsp olive oil (5ml)
- 1 tbsp tahini (15g)
- 1 tsp lemon juice (5ml)
- 1/4 tsp garlic powder (0.5g)
- 1/4 tsp black pepper (1g)
- 1/8 tsp salt (0.5g)

Instructions:

1. Cook freekeh according to package instructions.
2. Toss Brussels sprouts with olive oil, salt, and pepper. Roast at 400°F (200°C) for 20 minutes.
3. In a small bowl, whisk together tahini, lemon juice, garlic powder, and a splash of warm water.
4. Serve freekeh topped with roasted Brussels sprouts and drizzle with tahini sauce.

Nutritional Facts (Per Serving): Calories: 490 | Carbohydrates: 27g | Protein: 22g | Fat: 19g | Sugar: 3g | Fiber: 8g | Sodium: 520mg

Glycemic Index: Freekeh: 43 | Brussels sprouts: 15 | Tahini: 35

Quinoa Bowl with Sautéed Swiss Chard and Poached Egg

Prep: 10 minutes | Cook: 15 minutes | Serves: 1

Ingredients:

- 1/4 cup quinoa (45g)
- 1 cup chopped Swiss chard (40g)
- 1 egg, poached (50g)
- 1 tsp olive oil (5ml)
- 1/2 clove garlic, minced (2g)
- 1 tbsp fresh parsley, chopped (5g)
- Salt and pepper to taste

Instructions:

1. Cook quinoa according to instructions.
2. Sauté garlic and Swiss chard in olive oil until wilted (3–4 min).
3. Poach the egg in simmering water for 3–4 minutes.
4. Serve quinoa topped with greens, poached egg, and parsley.

Nutritional Facts (Per Serving): Calories: 475 | Carbohydrates: 23g | Protein: 21g | Fat: 18g | Sugar: 2g | Fiber: 5g | Sodium: 430mg

Glycemic Index: Quinoa: 53 | Swiss chard: 15 | Egg: 0

Amaranth and Mushroom Bowl with Herb Yogurt Sauce

Prep: 15 minutes | Cook: 25 minutes | Serves: 1

Ingredients:

- 1/4 cup amaranth (45g)
- 1/2 cup mushrooms, sliced (75g)
- 1 tbsp plain Greek yogurt (30g)
- 1/2 tsp olive oil (2ml)
- 1/2 tsp lemon juice (2.5ml)
- 1/4 tsp dried thyme (0.5g)
- Salt and pepper to taste

Instructions:

1. Cook amaranth in water until soft (15–20 min).
2. Sauté mushrooms in olive oil and thyme for 5–6 minutes.
3. Mix yogurt with lemon juice, salt, and pepper.
4. Assemble bowl with amaranth, mushrooms, and a dollop of herb yogurt.

Nutritional Facts (Per Serving): Calories: 485 | Carbohydrates: 25g | Protein: 22g | Fat: 17g | Sugar: 3g | Fiber: 4g | Sodium: 400mg

Glycemic Index: Amaranth: 47 | Mushrooms: 15 | Yogurt: 10

Teff Bowl with Roasted Carrot and Chickpeas

Prep: 15 minutes | **Cook:** 25 minutes | **Serves:** 1

Ingredients:

- 1/4 cup teff grain (45g)
- 1/2 cup diced carrot (60g)
- 1/4 cup canned chickpeas, rinsed (60g)
- 1 tsp olive oil (5ml)
- 1/2 tsp ground cumin (1g)
- 1/4 tsp black pepper (1g)
- 1/8 tsp salt (0.5g)

Instructions:

1. Cook teff in water for 15–20 minutes until soft.
2. Toss carrots and chickpeas with olive oil, cumin, salt, and pepper.
3. Roast at 400°F (200°C) for 20 minutes.
4. Serve roasted mix over teff.

Nutritional Facts (Per Serving): Calories: 488 | Carbohydrates: 26g | Protein: 21g | Fat: 17g | Sugar: 4g | Fiber: 6g | Sodium: 410mg

Glycemic Index: Teff: 57 (medium–low, in small portions) | Carrot: 47 | Chickpeas: 28

Barley Bowl with Grilled Tofu and Red Cabbage

Prep: 15 minutes | **Cook:** 20 minutes | **Serves:** 1

Ingredients:

- 1/4 cup pearl barley (50g)
- 1/2 cup red cabbage, shredded (40g)
- 1/2 cup firm tofu, cubed and grilled (100g)
- 1/2 tbsp sesame oil (7ml)
- 1 tsp soy sauce, low sodium (5ml)
- 1/4 tsp garlic powder (0.5g)
- 1/8 tsp black pepper (0.5g)

Instructions:

1. Cook barley according to instructions.
2. Grill tofu with soy sauce and garlic powder (4–5 min per side).
3. Sauté cabbage in sesame oil for 3–4 min.
4. Serve barley topped with tofu and cabbage.

Nutritional Facts (Per Serving): Calories: 480 | Carbohydrates: 24g | Protein: 23g | Fat: 17g | Sugar: 2g | Fiber: 6g | Sodium: 420mg

Glycemic Index: Barley: 28 | Tofu: 15 | Red cabbage: 15

Buckwheat Bowl with Smoked Salmon and Avocado

Prep: 10 minutes | **Cook:** 15 minutes | **Serves:** 1

Ingredients:

- 1/4 cup buckwheat groats (45g)
- 2 oz smoked salmon (60g)
- 1/4 avocado, sliced (50g)
- 1 tbsp lemon juice (15ml)
- 1 tsp olive oil (5ml)
- 1 tbsp fresh dill, chopped (5g)
- Black pepper to taste

Instructions:

1. Cook buckwheat as directed.
2. In a bowl, layer buckwheat, smoked salmon, and avocado.
3. Drizzle with olive oil and lemon juice. Sprinkle with dill and pepper.

Nutritional Facts (Per Serving): Calories: 495 | Carbohydrates: 22g | Protein: 24g | Fat: 20g | Sugar: 1g | Fiber: 5g | Sodium: 480mg

Glycemic Index: Buckwheat: 49 | Salmon: 0 | Avocado: 15

Quinoa and Black Bean Bowl with Cilantro-Lime Yogurt

Prep: 15 minutes | **Cook:** 20 minutes | **Serves:** 1

Ingredients:

- 1/4 cup quinoa (45g)
- 1/4 cup canned black beans, rinsed (60g)
- 1/4 cup chopped red bell pepper (40g)
- 1 tbsp plain Greek yogurt (30g)
- 1 tsp lime juice (5ml)
- 1 tbsp fresh cilantro, chopped (5g)
- Salt and pepper to taste

Instructions:

1. Cook quinoa according to package directions.
2. In a bowl, combine cooked quinoa, beans, and bell pepper.
3. In a separate bowl, mix yogurt, lime juice, and cilantro.
4. Serve yogurt dressing over the grain bowl.

Nutritional Facts (Per Serving): Calories: 486 | Carbohydrates: 25g | Protein: 23g | Fat: 18g | Sugar: 3g | Fiber: 7g | Sodium: 440mg

Glycemic Index: Quinoa: 53 | Black beans: 30 | Bell pepper: 15

Barley Bowl with Roasted Fennel and Chicken

Prep: 15 minutes | **Cook:** 25 minutes | **Serves:** 1

Ingredients:

- 1/4 cup pearl barley (50g)
- 4 oz grilled chicken breast, sliced (115g)
- 1/2 cup fennel bulb, sliced (50g)
- 1 tsp olive oil (5ml)
- 1/2 tsp lemon zest (1g)
- Salt and pepper to taste

Instructions:

1. Cook barley until tender.
2. Toss fennel with olive oil, salt, and pepper. Roast at 400°F (200°C) for 20 minutes.
3. Grill chicken until cooked through.
4. Assemble barley, chicken, and fennel in a bowl. Garnish with lemon zest.

Nutritional Facts (Per Serving): Calories: 480 | Carbohydrates: 24g | Protein: 24g | Fat: 18g | Sugar: 3g | Fiber: 4g | Sodium: 430mg

Glycemic Index: Barley: 28 | Chicken: 0 | Fennel: 15

Spelt Bowl with Sautéed Kale and Poached Egg

Prep: 10 minutes | **Cook:** 20 minutes | **Serves:** 1

Ingredients:

- 1/4 cup spelt grain (45g)
- 1 cup chopped kale (30g)
- 1 large egg, poached (50g)
- 1 tsp olive oil (5ml)
- 1/2 clove garlic, minced (2g)
- 1/8 tsp salt (0.5g)
- 1/4 tsp black pepper (1g)

Instructions:

1. Cook spelt in water for 20 minutes until soft.
2. Sauté kale and garlic in olive oil until wilted.
3. Poach the egg separately.
4. Assemble the bowl: spelt base, sautéed kale, and poached egg on top. Season to taste.

Nutritional Facts (Per Serving): Calories: 478 | Carbohydrates: 23g | Protein: 21g | Fat: 18g | Sugar: 2g | Fiber: 5g | Sodium: 410mg

Glycemic Index: Spelt: 44 | Kale: 15 | Egg: 0

Wholesome Casseroles for Lasting Energy

Zucchini Lasagna with Ground Turkey and Ricotta

Prep: 20 minutes | Cook: 40 minutes | Serves: 2

Ingredients:

- 2 medium zucchinis, sliced lengthwise (300g)
- 6 oz ground turkey (170g)
- 1/2 cup ricotta cheese (120g)
- 1 cup marinara sauce, no sugar added (240ml)
- 1 small onion, diced (70g)
- 1 tbsp olive oil (15ml)
- 1 tsp dried oregano (2g)
- 1/4 cup shredded mozzarella (30g)
- Salt and pepper to taste

Instructions:

1. Preheat the oven to 375°F (190°C).
2. Heat olive oil in a pan over medium heat. Add onion and ground turkey, cook until browned, about 5-7 minutes. Stir in marinara sauce and oregano.
3. In a baking dish, layer zucchini slices, ground turkey mixture, and ricotta. Repeat layers, ending with zucchini on top.
4. Sprinkle with shredded mozzarella. Bake for 30 minutes or until golden and bubbly.
5. Let cool for 5 minutes before serving.

Nutritional Facts (Per Serving): Calories: 500 | Carbohydrates: 20g | Protein: 24g | Fat: 20g | Fiber: 5g | Sugar: 7g | Sodium: 600mg

Glycemic Index: Zucchini: Low (GI = 15) | Ricotta: Low (GI = 27)

Eggplant Moussaka with Ground Beef and Parmesan

Prep: 20 minutes | Cook: 45 minutes | Serves: 2

Ingredients:

- 1 medium eggplant, sliced (300g)
- 6 oz ground beef, lean (170g)
- 1/2 cup tomato sauce, no sugar added (120ml)
- 1 small onion, diced (70g)
- 1/4 cup grated Parmesan cheese (30g)
- 1 tbsp olive oil (15ml)
- 1 tsp ground cinnamon (2g)
- 1 egg, beaten (50g)
- Salt and pepper to taste

Instructions:

1. Preheat oven to 375°F (190°C).
2. Brush eggplant slices with olive oil and roast in the oven for 20 minutes until tender.
3. In a pan, sauté onion and ground beef until browned, about 5-7 minutes. Stir in tomato sauce and cinnamon, simmer for 10 minutes.
4. In a baking dish, layer roasted eggplant, beef mixture, and beaten egg. Top with Parmesan cheese.
5. Bake for 25 minutes until golden and set.

Nutritional Facts (Per Serving): Calories: 500 | Carbohydrates: 16g | Protein: 25g | Fat: 20g | Fiber: 4g | Sugar: 5g | Sodium: 650mg

Glycemic Index: Eggplant: Low (GI = 15) | Parmesan: Low (GI = 27)

Spinach and Feta Crustless Quiche with Almond Flour

Prep: 15 minutes | Cook: 30 minutes | Serves: 2

Ingredients:

- 2 cups fresh spinach, chopped (60g)
- 4 large eggs (200g)
- 1/4 cup almond flour (30g)
- 1/4 cup crumbled feta cheese (30g)
- 1 tbsp olive oil (15ml)
- 1 clove garlic, minced (3g)
- Salt and pepper to taste

Instructions:

1. Preheat oven to 350°F (175°C).
2. Heat olive oil in a pan over medium heat. Add garlic and spinach, cook until wilted, about 2 minutes.
3. In a bowl, whisk eggs, almond flour, and feta cheese. Stir in cooked spinach.
4. Pour mixture into a greased baking dish and bake for 25-30 minutes until set.
5. Let cool for a few minutes before serving.

Nutritional Facts (Per Serving): Calories: 500 | Carbohydrates: 10g | Protein: 22g | Fat: 20g | Fiber: 3g | Sugar: 2g | Sodium: 600mg

Glycemic Index: Spinach: Low (GI = 15) | Feta: Low (GI = 30) | Almond Flour: Low (GI = 1)

Chicken and Cauliflower Rice Casserole with Broccoli

Prep: 15 minutes | Cook: 25 minutes | Serves: 2

Ingredients:

- 6 oz chicken breast, cooked and shredded (170g)
- 1 cup cauliflower rice (150g)
- 1 cup broccoli florets (150g)
- 1/2 cup shredded cheddar cheese (60g)
- 1 small onion, diced (70g)
- 1 tbsp olive oil (15ml)
- 1/2 cup low sodium chicken broth (120ml)
- 1 tsp garlic powder (2g)
- Salt and pepper to taste

Instructions:

1. Preheat oven to 375°F (190°C).
2. Heat olive oil in a pan, add onion and cook until softened, about 5 minutes.
3. Stir in cauliflower rice, chicken, broccoli, chicken broth, and garlic powder. Cook for 5 minutes.
4. Transfer mixture to a baking dish, top with shredded cheddar cheese.
5. Bake for 15-20 minutes until cheese is melted and bubbly.

Nutritional Facts (Per Serving): Calories: 500 | Carbohydrates: 15g | Protein: 25g | Fat: 20g | Fiber: 6g | Sugar: 4g | Sodium: 600mg

Glycemic Index: Cauliflower: Low (GI = 15) | Broccoli: Low (GI = 15)

Zucchini and Mushroom Lasagna with Ricotta and Mozzarella

Prep: 20 minutes | Cook: 40 minutes | Serves: 2

Ingredients:

- 2 medium zucchinis, sliced lengthwise (300g)
- 1 cup mushrooms, sliced (150g)
- 1/2 cup ricotta cheese (120g)
- 1/2 cup marinara sauce, no sugar added (120ml)
- 1/4 cup shredded mozzarella (30g)
- 1 tbsp olive oil (15ml)
- 1 tsp dried oregano (2g)
- Salt and pepper to taste

Instructions:

1. Preheat oven to 375°F (190°C).
2. Heat olive oil in a pan, sauté mushrooms until softened, about 5 minutes.
3. In a baking dish, layer zucchini slices, sautéed mushrooms, ricotta cheese, and marinara sauce. Repeat layers, ending with zucchini on top.
4. Top with shredded mozzarella and bake for 30-35 minutes until golden and bubbly.

Nutritional Facts (Per Serving): Calories: 500 | Carbohydrates: 18g | Protein: 22g | Fat: 20g | Fiber: 5g | Sugar: 6g | Sodium: 600mg

Glycemic Index: Zucchini: Low (GI = 15) | Ricotta: Low (GI = 27) | Mozzarella: Low (GI = 0)

Ground Turkey and Kale Casserole with Almond Crust

Prep: 15 minutes | Cook: 30 minutes | Serves: 2

Ingredients:

- 6 oz ground turkey (170g)
- 2 cups kale, chopped (60g)
- 1/2 cup almond flour (60g)
- 1 small onion, diced (70g)
- 1 tbsp olive oil (15ml)
- 1 egg, beaten (50g)
- 1 tsp paprika (2g)
- Salt and pepper to taste

Instructions:

1. Preheat oven to 350°F (175°C).
2. Heat olive oil in a pan, cook ground turkey and onion until browned, about 7 minutes. Stir in chopped kale and cook until wilted, about 3 minutes.
3. In a bowl, mix almond flour, beaten egg, paprika, salt, and pepper to form the almond crust mixture.
4. Transfer turkey mixture to a baking dish, spread almond crust mixture over the top.
5. Bake for 20 minutes until golden and set.

Nutritional Facts (Per Serving): Calories: 500 | Carbohydrates: 12g | Protein: 23g | Fat: 20g | Fiber: 6g | Sugar: 3g | Sodium: 550mg

Glycemic Index: Kale: Low (GI = 15) | Almond Flour: Low (GI = 1)

Mushroom and Ground Beef Casserole with Cauliflower

Prep: 15 minutes | Cook: 30 minutes | Serves: 2

Ingredients:

- 6 oz ground beef, lean (170g)
- 1 cup cauliflower florets, chopped (150g)
- 1 cup mushrooms, sliced (150g)
- 1 small onion, diced (70g)
- 1 tbsp olive oil (15ml)
- 1/2 cup shredded cheddar cheese (60g)
- 1/2 cup low sodium beef broth (120ml)
- 1 tsp dried thyme (2g)
- Salt and pepper to taste

Instructions:

1. Preheat oven to 375°F (190°C).
2. Brown beef in oil (7 min), add onion, mushrooms, thyme — cook 5 min.
3. Stir in cauliflower and beef broth, cook for another 5 minutes.
4. Transfer mixture to a baking dish, sprinkle with cheddar cheese, and bake for 15 minutes until golden and bubbly.

Nutritional Facts (Per Serving): Calories: 500 | Carbohydrates: 12g | Protein: 24g | Fat: 20g | Fiber: 4g | Sugar: 3g | Sodium: 600mg

Glycemic Index: Cauliflower: Low (GI = 15) | Mushrooms: Low (GI = 15)

Spaghetti Squash Casserole with Chicken and Alfredo Sauce

Prep: 20 minutes | Cook: 40 minutes | Serves: 2

Ingredients:

- 1 small spaghetti squash (600g)
- 6 oz chicken breast, cooked and shredded (170g)
- 1/2 cup Alfredo sauce, low carb (120ml)
- 1 cup spinach, fresh (30g)
- 1 tbsp olive oil (15ml)
- 1/4 cup grated Parmesan cheese (30g)
- 1 tsp garlic powder (2g)
- Salt and pepper to taste

Instructions:

1. Preheat oven to 375°F (190°C). Cut spaghetti squash in half, scoop out seeds, and roast for 30-35 minutes. Scrape out the strands.
2. In a pan, heat olive oil, add spinach and cook until wilted, about 2 minutes.
3. In a bowl, mix spaghetti squash strands, shredded chicken, spinach, Alfredo sauce, garlic powder, salt, and pepper.
4. Transfer to a baking dish, top with Parmesan cheese, and bake for 10 minutes until bubbly.

Nutritional Facts (Per Serving): Calories: 500 | Carbohydrates: 18g | Protein: 25g | Fat: 20g | Fiber: 5g | Sugar: 5g | Sodium: 650mg

Glycemic Index: Spaghetti Squash: Low (GI = 41) | Parmesan: Low (GI = 27)

Butternut Squash and Zucchini Lasagna with Turkey and Ricotta

Prep: 20 minutes | Cook: 40 minutes | Serves: 2

Ingredients:

- 1 small butternut squash, sliced (300g)
- 1 medium zucchini, sliced lengthwise (150g)
- 6 oz ground turkey (170g)
- 1/2 cup ricotta cheese (120g)
- 1/2 cup marinara sauce, no sugar added (120ml)
- 1/4 cup shredded mozzarella (30g)
- 1 tbsp olive oil (15ml)
- 1 tsp dried oregano (2g)
- Salt and pepper to taste

Instructions:

1. Preheat oven to 375°F (190°C).
2. Heat olive oil in a pan, cook ground turkey until browned, about 7 minutes. Stir in marinara sauce and oregano.
3. In a baking dish, layer butternut squash, zucchini slices, turkey mixture, and ricotta cheese. Repeat layers, ending with zucchini on top.
4. Sprinkle with mozzarella and bake for 30 minutes until golden and bubbly.

Nutritional Facts (Per Serving): Calories: 500 | Carbohydrates: 25g | Protein: 24g | Fat: 20g | Fiber: 6g | Sugar: 7g | Sodium: 600mg

Glycemic Index: Butternut Squash: Medium (GI = 51) | Zucchini: Low (GI = 15)

Italian-Style Stuffed Zucchini Boats with Ricotta and Spinach

Prep: 15 minutes | Cook: 25 minutes | Serves: 2

Ingredients:

- 2 medium zucchinis, halved lengthwise (300g)
- 1/2 cup ricotta cheese (120g)
- 1 cup spinach, fresh, chopped (30g)
- 1 small onion, diced (70g)
- 1 clove garlic, minced (3g)
- 1 tbsp olive oil (15ml)
- 1/4 cup shredded mozzarella (30g)
- 1 tsp dried basil (2g)
- Salt and pepper to taste

Instructions:

1. Preheat oven to 375°F (190°C).
2. Scoop out the centers of the zucchini halves to create boats.
3. Heat olive oil in a pan, sauté onion, garlic, and spinach for 3-4 minutes until softened.
4. In a bowl, mix ricotta, sautéed spinach, basil, salt, and pepper. Fill zucchini boats with the mixture.
5. Top with shredded mozzarella and bake for 20-25 minutes until golden and bubbly.

Nutritional Facts (Per Serving): Calories: 500 | Carbohydrates: 14g | Protein: 22g | Fat: 20g | Fiber: 5g | Sugar: 5g | Sodium: 600mg

Glycemic Index: Zucchini: Low (GI = 15) | Ricotta: Low (GI = 27)

Spiced Ground Beef Stuffed Eggplants with Almonds and Herbs

Prep: 20 minutes | Cook: 35 minutes | Serves: 2

Ingredients:

- 2 small eggplants, halved and hollowed out (300g)
- 6 oz ground beef, lean (170g)
- 1 small onion, diced (70g)
- 2 tbsp almonds, chopped (20g)
- 1 clove garlic, minced (3g)
- 1 tbsp olive oil (15ml)
- 1 tsp ground cumin (2g)
- 2 tbsp fresh parsley, chopped (10g)
- Salt and pepper to taste

Instructions:

1. Preheat oven to 375°F (190°C).
2. Brush eggplant halves with olive oil and roast for 20 minutes.
3. Heat olive oil in a pan, sauté onion and garlic until softened, then add ground beef and cumin. Cook until browned, about 7 minutes. Stir in almonds and parsley.
4. Stuff the eggplant halves with the beef mixture and bake for an additional 15 minutes.

Nutritional Facts (Per Serving): Calories: 500 | Carbohydrates: 15g | Protein: 24g | Fat: 20g | Fiber: 5g | Sugar: 4g | Sodium: 600mg

Glycemic Index: Eggplant: Low (GI = 15) | Almonds: Low (GI = 0)

Zucchini and Mushroom Stir-Fry with Garlic and Almonds

Prep: 10 minutes | Cook: 15 minutes | Serves: 2

Ingredients:

- 2 medium zucchinis, sliced (300g)
- 1 cup mushrooms, sliced (150g)
- 1 clove garlic, minced (3g)
- 2 tbsp almonds, sliced (20g)
- 1 tbsp olive oil (15ml)
- 1 tsp soy sauce, low sodium (5ml)
- Salt and pepper to taste

Instructions:

1. Heat olive oil in a pan over medium heat. Add garlic and sauté for 1 minute.
2. Add zucchini and mushrooms, stir-fry for 5-7 minutes until tender.
3. Stir in soy sauce, almonds, salt, and pepper. Cook for another 2 minutes. Serve warm.

Nutritional Facts (Per Serving): Calories: 500 | Carbohydrates: 18g | Protein: 22g | Fat: 20g | Fiber: 6g | Sugar: 5g | Sodium: 600mg

Glycemic Index: Zucchini: Low (GI = 15) | Mushrooms: Low (GI = 15) | Almonds: Low (GI = 0)

Broccoli and Turkey Breakfast Bake with Cheddar

Prep: 10 minutes | Cook: 30 minutes | Serves: 1

Ingredients:

- 2 large eggs (100g)
- 3 oz ground turkey (85g)
- 1/2 cup broccoli florets, chopped (75g)
- 1/4 cup shredded cheddar cheese (30g)
- 1 tbsp onion, minced (15g)
- 1 tsp olive oil (5ml)
- 1/4 tsp garlic powder (0.5g)
- Salt and pepper to taste

Instructions:

1. Preheat oven to 375°F (190°C).
2. In a pan, sauté ground turkey and onion in olive oil until browned.
3. Whisk eggs with garlic powder, salt, and pepper.
4. In a small baking dish, combine turkey, broccoli, and egg mixture. Top with cheddar.
5. Bake for 25–30 minutes until set.

Nutritional Facts (Per Serving): Calories: 485 | Carbohydrates: 6g | Protein: 24g | Fat: 20g | Sugar: 2g | Fiber: 2g | Sodium: 460mg

Glycemic Index: Broccoli: 15 | Egg: 0 | Cheddar: 0

Eggplant & Chicken Casserole with Herb Yogurt

Prep: 15 minutes | Cook: 30 minutes | Serves: 1

Ingredients:

- 1/2 medium eggplant, sliced (150g)
- 4 oz ground chicken (115g)
- 2 tbsp plain Greek yogurt (30g)
- 1/2 tsp dried oregano (1g)
- 1/4 cup shredded mozzarella (30g)
- 1 tsp olive oil (5ml)
- Salt and pepper to taste

Instructions:

1. Preheat oven to 375°F (190°C).
2. Sauté ground chicken with salt and pepper until browned.
3. Grill or sauté eggplant slices lightly in olive oil.
4. In a small dish, layer eggplant, chicken, and mozzarella.
5. Top with yogurt mixed with oregano. Bake for 20 minutes.

Nutritional Facts (Per Serving): Calories: 495 | Carbohydrates: 8g | Protein: 24g | Fat: 21g | Sugar: 3g | Fiber: 3g | Sodium: 470mg

Glycemic Index: Eggplant: 15 | Yogurt: 10 | Mozzarella: 0

Cabbage and Tofu Bake with Almond Crumble

Prep: 10 minutes | Cook: 25 minutes | Serves: 1

Ingredients:

- 1 cup shredded white cabbage (70g)
- 1/2 cup firm tofu, crumbled (100g)
- 1 tbsp almond flour (10g)
- 1 tbsp sliced almonds (10g)
- 1 large egg (50g)
- 1 tsp olive oil (5ml)
- 1/2 tsp mustard (2g)
- Salt and black pepper to taste

Instructions:

1. Preheat oven to 350°F (175°C).
2. In a bowl, mix cabbage, tofu, beaten egg, mustard, salt, and pepper.
3. Place mixture in a greased baking dish.
4. Top with almond flour and sliced almonds.
5. Bake for 25 minutes until firm and lightly golden.

Nutritional Facts (Per Serving): Calories: 478 | Carbohydrates: 7g | Protein: 23g | Fat: 19g | Sugar: 2g | Fiber: 3g | Sodium: 430mg

Glycemic Index: Cabbage: 15 | Tofu: 15 | Almond flour: 1

Cauliflower and Sardine Casserole with Lemon-Parsley Crust

Prep: 12 minutes | Cook: 25 minutes | Serves: 1

Ingredients:

- 1 cup cauliflower florets, chopped (150g)
- 1 small can sardines in water, drained (90g)
- 1 egg (50g)
- 1 tsp lemon juice (5ml)
- 1 tbsp almond flour (10g)
- 1 tbsp chopped parsley (5g)
- Salt and black pepper to taste

Instructions:

1. Preheat oven to 375°F (190°C).
2. Steam cauliflower for 5–6 minutes until tender.
3. In a bowl, mix cauliflower, sardines, egg, lemon juice, salt, and pepper.
4. Transfer to a baking dish. Mix almond flour and parsley, sprinkle on top.
5. Bake for 20–25 minutes until golden.

Nutritional Facts (Per Serving): Calories: 490 | Carbohydrates: 6g | Protein: 25g | Fat: 20g | Sugar: 1g | Fiber: 2g | Sodium: 460mg

Glycemic Index: Cauliflower: 15 | Sardines: 0 | Almond flour: 1

Tofu and Mushroom Crustless Pie with Herbs

Prep: 10 minutes | Cook: 30 minutes | Serves: 1

Ingredients:

- 1/2 cup firm tofu, mashed (100g)
- 1/2 cup mushrooms, diced (75g)
- 2 large eggs (100g)
- 1/4 cup chopped leek (40g)
- 1 tsp olive oil (5ml)
- 1/2 tsp thyme (0.5g)
- Salt and pepper to taste

Instructions:

1. Preheat oven to 375°F (190°C).
2. Sauté leek and mushrooms in olive oil for 4–5 minutes.
3. In a bowl, mix eggs, tofu, thyme, salt, and pepper. Stir in vegetables.
4. Pour into a greased dish and bake for 25–30 minutes until set.

Nutritional Facts (Per Serving): Calories: 475 | Carbohydrates: 5g | Protein: 23g | Fat: 19g | Sugar: 2g | Fiber: 2g | Sodium: 420mg

Glycemic Index: Tofu: 15 | Mushroom: 15 | Egg: 0

Chard and Ricotta Bake with Tomato Slices

Prep: 10 minutes | Cook: 30 minutes | Serves: 1

Ingredients:

- 1 cup Swiss chard, chopped (40g)
- 1/2 cup ricotta cheese (120g)
- 1 egg (50g)
- 1 medium tomato, sliced (120g)
- 1 tsp olive oil (5ml)
- 1/2 tsp dried basil (0.5g)
- Salt and pepper to taste

Instructions:

1. Preheat oven to 375°F (190°C).
2. In a bowl, mix ricotta, chopped chard, beaten egg, basil, salt, and pepper.
3. Pour into a baking dish. Lay tomato slices on top, brush with olive oil.
4. Bake for 25–30 minutes until golden and set.

Nutritional Facts (Per Serving): Calories: 480 | Carbohydrates: 8g | Protein: 22g | Fat: 20g | Sugar: 3g | Fiber: 2g | Sodium: 430mg

Glycemic Index: Chard: 15 | Ricotta: 27 | Tomato: 30

Crustless Zucchini Pie with Goat Cheese and Dill

Prep: 10 minutes | Cook: 30 minutes | Serves: 1

Ingredients:

- 1 small zucchini, grated (150g)
- 2 large eggs (100g)
- 2 tbsp goat cheese, crumbled (30g)
- 1 tbsp chopped fresh dill (5g)
- 1 tsp olive oil (5ml)
- Salt and black pepper to taste

Instructions:

1. Preheat oven to 375°F (190°C).
2. Grate zucchini, squeeze excess moisture.
3. In a bowl, mix eggs, goat cheese, dill, salt, and pepper. Stir in zucchini.
4. Pour into a greased small baking dish.
5. Bake for 25–30 minutes until golden and firm.

Nutritional Facts (Per Serving): Calories: 475 | Carbohydrates: 6g | Protein: 22g | Fat: 20g | Sugar: 2g | Fiber: 2g | Sodium: 420mg

Glycemic Index: Zucchini: 15 | Goat Cheese: 0 | Eggs: 0

Baked Cabbage and Ground Beef Gratin with Cheese

Prep: 15 minutes | Cook: 25 minutes | Serves: 1

Ingredients:

- 1 cup shredded cabbage (70g)
- 4 oz lean ground beef (115g)
- 1/4 cup shredded mozzarella (30g)
- 1 tbsp chopped onion (15g)
- 1/2 tsp garlic powder (0.5g)
- 1 tsp olive oil (5ml)
- Salt and pepper to taste

Instructions:

1. Preheat oven to 375°F (190°C).
2. Sauté beef and onion in olive oil, add garlic powder, salt, and pepper.
3. In a baking dish, layer cabbage and beef mixture.
4. Top with shredded mozzarella.
5. Bake for 20–25 minutes until bubbly and golden.

Nutritional Facts (Per Serving): Calories: 495 | Carbohydrates: 7g | Protein: 24g | Fat: 20g | Sugar: 3g | Fiber: 2g | Sodium: 440mg

Glycemic Index: Cabbage: 15 | Beef: 0 | Mozzarella: 0

Brussels Sprouts and Chicken Casserole with Almond Crust

Prep: 15 minutes | Cook: 30 minutes | Serves: 1

Ingredients:

- 1/2 cup cooked shredded chicken breast (85g)
- 1 cup Brussels sprouts, halved (120g)
- 1 large egg (50g)
- 1 tbsp almond flour (10g)
- 1/2 clove garlic, minced (2g)
- 1 tsp olive oil (5ml)
- Salt and pepper to taste

Instructions:

1. Preheat oven to 375°F (190°C).
2. Steam or roast Brussels sprouts for 10 minutes.
3. In a bowl, mix chicken, sprouts, egg, garlic, salt, and pepper.
4. Transfer to baking dish. Top with almond flour and drizzle with olive oil.
5. Bake for 20 minutes until golden.

Nutritional Facts (Per Serving): Calories: 478 | Carbohydrates: 8g | Protein: 24g | Fat: 19g | Sugar: 2g | Fiber: 3g | Sodium: 430mg

Glycemic Index: Brussels sprouts: 15 | Chicken: 0 | Almond flour: 1

Protein-Packed Meat Dishes

French-Style Baked Meat

Prep: 15 minutes | Cook: 35 minutes | Serves: 2

Ingredients:

- 8 oz pork loin, thinly sliced (225g)
- 1 medium onion, sliced (70g)
- 1 small tomato, sliced (100g)
- 1/4 cup grated cheese (30g)
- 2 tbsp sour cream, low fat (30ml)
- 1 tbsp olive oil (15ml)
- 1 tsp dried oregano (2g)
- Salt and pepper to taste

Instructions:

1. Preheat oven to 375°F (190°C).
2. Layer pork slices in a greased baking dish. Season with salt, pepper, and oregano.
3. Top with sliced onions and tomatoes, then spread sour cream over the top.
4. Sprinkle with grated cheese and bake for 30-35 minutes until golden and bubbly.

Nutritional Facts (Per Serving): Calories: 500 | Carbohydrates: 8g | Protein: 24g | Fat: 20g | Fiber: 2g | Sugar: 4g | Sodium: 600mg

Glycemic Index: Tomato: Low (GI = 15) | Onion: Low (GI = 10)

Grilled Turkey Tenderloin with Roasted Vegetables

Prep: 15 minutes | Cook: 25 minutes | Serves: 2

Ingredients:

- 6 oz turkey tenderloin (170g)
- 1 small zucchini, chopped (150g)
- 1 small red bell pepper, chopped (100g)
- 1 small onion, chopped (70g)
- 1 tbsp olive oil (15ml)
- 1 tsp dried thyme (2g)
- Salt and pepper to taste

Instructions:

1. Preheat grill to medium heat.
2. Season turkey tenderloin with salt, pepper, and thyme. Grill for 8-10 minutes per side until fully cooked.
3. Toss zucchini, bell pepper, and onion with olive oil, salt, and pepper. Roast in a preheated oven at 400°F (200°C) for 20 minutes.
4. Serve the grilled turkey with roasted vegetables.

Nutritional Facts (Per Serving): Calories: 500 | Carbohydrates: 18g | Protein: 25g | Fat: 19g | Fiber: 6g | Sugar: 5g | Sodium: 600mg

Glycemic Index: Zucchini: Low (GI = 15) | Bell Pepper: Low (GI = 15)

Stuffed Turkey Roll with Spinach & Feta

Prep: 20 minutes | Cook: 30 minutes | Serves: 2

Ingredients:

- 6 oz turkey breast, pounded thin (170g)
- 1/2 cup spinach, fresh (30g)
- 1/4 cup feta cheese, crumbled (30g)
- 1 small zucchini, sliced (150g)
- 1 tbsp olive oil (15ml)
- 1 clove garlic, minced (3g)
- Salt and pepper to taste

Instructions:

1. Preheat oven to 375°F (190°C).
2. Spread spinach and feta evenly over turkey breast. Roll up tightly and secure with toothpicks.
3. Bake for 25-30 minutes until fully cooked.
4. Meanwhile, heat olive oil in a pan over medium heat, sauté zucchini and garlic for 5-7 minutes until tender.
5. Serve turkey roll with sautéed zucchini.

Nutritional Facts (Per Serving): Calories: 500 | Carbohydrates: 10g | Protein: 24g | Fat: 20g | Fiber: 4g | Sugar: 3g | Sodium: 600mg

Glycemic Index: Zucchini: Low (GI = 15) | Feta: Low (GI = 30)

Grilled Flank Steak with Quinoa and Roasted Brussels Sprouts

Prep: 15 minutes | Cook: 25 minutes | Serves: 2

Ingredients:

- 6 oz flank steak (170g)
- 1/2 cup quinoa, cooked (90g)
- 1 cup Brussels sprouts, halved (150g)
- 1 tbsp olive oil (15ml)
- 1 tsp garlic powder (2g)
- Salt and pepper to taste

Instructions:

1. Preheat grill to medium heat. Season flank steak with garlic powder, salt, and pepper. Grill for 4-5 minutes per side, then let rest for 5 minutes before slicing.
2. Toss Brussels sprouts with olive oil, salt, and pepper, and roast in the oven at 400°F (200°C) for 20 minutes.
3. Serve sliced flank steak with quinoa and roasted Brussels sprouts.

Nutritional Facts (Per Serving): Calories: 500 | Carbohydrates: 20g | Protein: 25g | Fat: 20g | Fiber: 6g | Sugar: 3g | Sodium: 600mg

Glycemic Index: Quinoa: Low (GI = 53) | Brussels Sprouts: Low (GI = 15)

Spinach and Ricotta-Stuffed Chicken Roll with Cauliflower Mash

Prep: 20 minutes | Cook: 30 minutes | Serves: 2

Ingredients:

- 6 oz chicken breast, pounded thin (170g)
- 1/2 cup ricotta cheese (120g)
- 1 cup spinach, fresh, chopped (30g)
- 1 small cauliflower, chopped (150g)
- 1 tbsp olive oil (15ml)
- 1 clove garlic, minced (3g)
- 1 tbsp unsalted butter (15g)
- Salt and pepper to taste

Instructions:

1. Preheat oven to 375°F (190°C).
2. Mix ricotta, spinach, garlic, salt, and pepper. Spread over chicken breast, roll up, and secure with toothpicks. Bake for 25-30 minutes until fully cooked.
3. Boil cauliflower until tender, about 10 minutes. Drain and mash with butter, salt, and pepper.
4. Serve chicken roll with cauliflower mash.

Nutritional Facts (Per Serving): Calories: 500 | Carbohydrates: 12g | Protein: 24g | Fat: 20g | Fiber: 5g | Sugar: 3g | Sodium: 600mg

Glycemic Index: Cauliflower: Low (GI = 15) | Ricotta: Low (GI = 27)

Balsamic Glazed Beef Tenderloin with Garlic Sautéed Kale

Prep: 15 minutes | Cook: 25 minutes | Serves: 2

Ingredients:

- 6 oz beef tenderloin (170g)
- 1 tbsp balsamic vinegar (15ml)
- 1 tbsp olive oil (15ml)
- 2 cups kale, chopped (60g)
- 2 cloves garlic, minced (6g)
- Salt and pepper to taste

Instructions:

1. Preheat oven to 400°F (200°C). Season beef tenderloin with salt and pepper. Sear in a hot pan with olive oil for 2-3 minutes per side, then transfer to the oven for 10-12 minutes.
2. In the last 5 minutes of cooking, brush tenderloin with balsamic vinegar. Let rest before slicing.
3. Sauté garlic in olive oil, add kale, and cook until wilted, about 5 minutes.
4. Serve sliced beef tenderloin with garlic sautéed kale.

Nutritional Facts (Per Serving): Calories: 500 | Carbohydrates: 10g | Protein: 25g | Fat: 20g | Fiber: 4g | Sugar: 5g | Sodium: 600mg

Glycemic Index: Kale: Low (GI = 15) | Balsamic Vinegar: Low (GI = 5)

Chicken Roulade with Goat Cheese & Tomatoes

Prep: 20 minutes | Cook: 25 minutes | Serves: 2

Ingredients:

- 6 oz chicken breast, pounded thin (170g)
- 2 tbsp goat cheese (30g)
- 2 tbsp sundried tomatoes, chopped (30g)
- 1 medium zucchini, spiralized (150g)
- 1 tbsp olive oil (15ml)
- 1 clove garlic, minced (3g)
- 1 tsp dried oregano (2g)
- Salt and pepper to taste

Instructions:

1. Preheat oven to 375°F (190°C).
2. Spread goat cheese and sundried tomatoes on the chicken breast, roll up and secure with toothpicks.
3. Bake for 20-25 minutes until fully cooked.
4. Heat olive oil in a pan, sauté garlic and zucchini noodles for 3-4 minutes.
5. Serve chicken roulade with zucchini noodles.

Nutritional Facts (Per Serving): Calories: 500 | Carbohydrates: 10g | Protein: 24g | Fat: 20g | Fiber: 3g | Sugar: 4g | Sodium: 600mg

Glycemic Index: Zucchini: Low (GI = 15) | Goat Cheese: Low (GI = 0)

Grilled Sirloin with Cauli Rice & Asparagus

Prep: 15 minutes | Cook: 20 minutes | Serves: 2

Ingredients:

- 6 oz sirloin steak (170g)
- 1 cup cauliflower rice (150g)
- 1 cup asparagus, trimmed (150g)
- 1 tbsp olive oil (15ml)
- 1 tsp garlic powder (2g)
- Salt and pepper to taste

Instructions:

1. Preheat grill to medium heat. Season steak with garlic powder, salt, and pepper. Grill for 4-5 minutes per side, then let rest for 5 minutes.
2. Toss asparagus with olive oil, salt, and pepper. Roast in a preheated oven at 400°F (200°C) for 15 minutes.
3. Sauté cauliflower rice in a pan for 5 minutes until tender.
4. Serve grilled steak with cauliflower rice and roasted asparagus.

Nutritional Facts (Per Serving): Calories: 500 | Carbohydrates: 12g | Protein: 25g | Fat: 20g | Fiber: 4g | Sugar: 3g | Sodium: 600mg

Glycemic Index: Cauliflower: Low (GI = 15) | Asparagus: Low (GI = 15)

Turkey Meatloaf Roll with Mushrooms

Prep: 20 minutes | Cook: 30 minutes | Serves: 2

Ingredients:

- 6 oz ground turkey (170g)
- 1 cup mushrooms, chopped (150g)
- 1/4 cup grated Parmesan cheese (30g)
- 1 small onion, diced (70g)
- 1 egg, beaten (50g)
- 1 cup broccoli florets (150g)
- 1 tbsp olive oil (15ml)
- 1 tsp dried thyme (2g)
- Salt and pepper to taste

Instructions:

1. Preheat oven to 375°F (190°C).
2. In a bowl, mix ground turkey, mushrooms, onion, Parmesan, egg, thyme, salt, and pepper. Shape into a roll and place in a baking dish.
3. Bake for 25-30 minutes until fully cooked.
4. Steam broccoli for 5 minutes, then drizzle with olive oil before serving.
5. Serve turkey meatloaf roll with steamed broccoli.

Nutritional Facts (Per Serving): Calories: 500 | Carbohydrates: 12g | Protein: 24g | Fat: 20g | Fiber: 4g | Sugar: 3g | Sodium: 600mg

Glycemic Index: Broccoli: Low (GI = 15) | Parmesan: Low (GI = 27)

Beef Roll with Spinach, Feta & Eggplant

Prep: 20 minutes | Cook: 30 minutes | Serves: 2

Ingredients:

- 6 oz beef flank steak, pounded thin (170g)
- 1/2 cup spinach, fresh, chopped (30g)
- 1/4 cup feta cheese, crumbled (30g)
- 1 medium eggplant, sliced (150g)
- 1 tbsp olive oil (15ml)
- 1 clove garlic, minced (3g)
- 1 tsp dried oregano (2g)
- Salt and pepper to taste

Instructions:

1. Preheat oven to 375°F (190°C).
2. Spread spinach and feta cheese over beef. Roll up and secure with toothpicks. Season with garlic, oregano, salt, and pepper.
3. Roast for 20-25 minutes until fully cooked.
4. Toss eggplant slices with olive oil, salt, and pepper, and roast alongside the beef for 20 minutes.
5. Serve beef roll with roasted eggplant.

Nutritional Facts (Per Serving): Calories: 500 | Carbohydrates: 12g | Protein: 24g | Fat: 20g | Fiber: 4g | Sugar: 5g | Sodium: 600mg

Glycemic Index: Eggplant: Low (GI = 15) | Feta: Low (GI = 30)

Pork Loin with Apple & Sage

Prep: 20 minutes | Cook: 40 minutes | Serves: 2

Ingredients:

- 6 oz pork loin, butterflied (170g)
- 1/2 apple, thinly sliced (75g)
- 1 tsp fresh sage, chopped (2g)
- 1 cup red cabbage, shredded (150g)
- 1 tbsp olive oil (15ml)
- 1 tbsp apple cider vinegar (15ml)
- 1 tsp low carb sweetener
- Salt and pepper to taste

Instructions:

1. Preheat oven to 375°F (190°C).
2. Lay apple slices and sage inside pork loin, roll up and secure with toothpicks. Roast for 25-30 minutes.
3. Meanwhile, heat olive oil in a pan and sauté cabbage for 5 minutes. Add apple cider vinegar, low carb sweetener, salt, and pepper. Simmer for 15 minutes until tender.
4. Serve pork loin with braised red cabbage.

Nutritional Facts (Per Serving): Calories: 500 | Carbohydrates: 18g | Protein: 24g | Fat: 19g | Fiber: 5g | Sugar: 7g | Sodium: 600mg

Glycemic Index: Apple: Medium (GI = 38) | Red Cabbage: Low (GI = 15)

Chicken Roll with Pesto & Mozzarella

Prep: 20 minutes | Cook: 30 minutes | Serves: 2

Ingredients:

- 6 oz chicken breast, pounded thin (170g)
- 2 tbsp pesto (30g)
- 1/4 cup shredded mozzarella (30g)
- 1 medium zucchini, spiralized into ribbons (150g)
- 1 tbsp olive oil (15ml)
- 1 clove garlic, minced (3g)
- Salt and pepper to taste

Instructions:

1. Preheat oven to 375°F (190°C).
2. Spread pesto and mozzarella over chicken breast, roll up and secure with toothpicks. Bake for 25-30 minutes until fully cooked.
3. Heat olive oil in a pan, sauté garlic and zucchini ribbons for 3-4 minutes until tender.
4. Serve chicken roll with zucchini ribbons.

Nutritional Facts (Per Serving): Calories: 500 | Carbohydrates: 10g | Protein: 25g | Fat: 20g | Fiber: 4g | Sugar: 3g | Sodium: 600mg

Glycemic Index: Zucchini: Low (GI = 15) | Mozzarella: Low (GI = 0)

Herb-Marinated Chicken Wings with Cauliflower Mash

Prep: 15 minutes | Cook: 35 minutes | Serves: 2

Ingredients:

- 6 chicken wings (300g)
- 1 small cauliflower, chopped (150g)
- 2 tbsp olive oil (30ml)
- 1 tsp dried thyme (2g)
- 1 tsp dried rosemary (2g)
- 1 clove garlic, minced (3g)
- 1 tbsp butter (15g)
- Salt and pepper to taste

Instructions:

1. Preheat oven to 400°F (200°C).
2. Marinate chicken wings in olive oil, garlic, thyme, rosemary, salt, and pepper. Roast for 30-35 minutes until crispy.
3. Boil cauliflower until tender, about 10 minutes. Drain and mash with butter, salt, and pepper.
4. Serve chicken wings with cauliflower mash.

Nutritional Facts (Per Serving): Calories: 500 | Carbohydrates: 10g | Protein: 24g | Fat: 20g | Fiber: 4g | Sugar: 3g | Sodium: 600mg

Glycemic Index: Cauliflower: Low (GI = 15)

Buffalo Chicken Wings with Cucumber and Celery Salad

Prep: 15 minutes | Cook: 30 minutes | Serves: 2

Ingredients:

- 6 chicken wings (300g)
- 2 tbsp hot sauce (30ml)
- 1 tbsp butter, melted (15g)
- 1 small cucumber, sliced (100g)
- 1 cup celery sticks (100g)
- 1 tbsp olive oil (15ml)
- 1 tsp apple cider vinegar (5ml)
- Salt and pepper to taste

Instructions:

1. Preheat oven to 400°F (200°C).
2. Toss chicken wings with melted butter and hot sauce. Roast for 25-30 minutes until crispy.
3. In a bowl, mix cucumber, celery, olive oil, vinegar, salt, and pepper for the salad.
4. Serve buffalo chicken wings with cucumber and celery salad.

Nutritional Facts (Per Serving): Calories: 500 | Carbohydrates: 12g | Protein: 23g | Fat: 20g | Fiber: 4g | Sugar: 2g | Sodium: 600mg

Glycemic Index: Cucumber: Low (GI = 15) | Celery: Low (GI = 15)

Low-Carb BBQ Chicken Drumsticks with Coleslaw and Avocado

Prep: 20 minutes | Cook: 30 minutes | Serves: 2

Ingredients:

- 4 chicken drumsticks (300g)
- 2 tbsp low-carb BBQ sauce (30ml)
- 1 cup shredded cabbage (100g)
- 1/2 small carrot, grated (50g)
- 1/2 avocado, sliced (75g)
- 1 tbsp olive oil (15ml)
- 1 tbsp apple cider vinegar (15ml)
- Salt and pepper to taste

Instructions:

1. Preheat oven to 400°F (200°C).
2. Brush chicken drumsticks with BBQ sauce and roast for 25-30 minutes.
3. In a bowl, mix shredded cabbage, carrot, olive oil, vinegar, salt, and pepper to make coleslaw.
4. Serve BBQ chicken drumsticks with coleslaw and avocado slices.

Nutritional Facts (Per Serving): Calories: 500 | Carbohydrates: 15g | Protein: 24g | Fat: 20g | Fiber: 6g | Sugar: 4g | Sodium: 600mg

Glycemic Index: Cabbage: Low (GI = 15) | Avocado: Low (GI = 15)

Rosemary Veal Chops with Steamed Broccolini

Prep: 10 minutes | **Cook:** 15 minutes | **Serves:** 1

Ingredients:

- 5 oz veal chop, boneless (140g)
- 1 cup broccolini, trimmed (100g)
- 1 tsp olive oil (5ml)
- 1/2 tsp fresh rosemary, chopped (1g)
- 1/2 clove garlic, minced (2g)
- Salt and pepper to taste

Instructions:

1. Rub veal chop with garlic, rosemary, salt, and pepper.
2. Sear in a hot skillet with olive oil for 3–4 minutes per side until browned and cooked through.
3. Steam broccolini for 5–6 minutes until tender.
4. Serve veal with broccolini on the side.

Nutritional Facts (Per Serving): Calories: 495 | Carbohydrates: 7g | Protein: 25g | Fat: 20g | Sugar: 2g | Fiber: 3g | Sodium: 440mg

Glycemic Index: Veal: 0 | Broccolini: 15

Spiced Lamb Patties with Mint Yogurt and Grilled Eggplant

Prep: 15 minutes | **Cook:** 20 minutes | **Serves:** 1

Ingredients:

- 4 oz ground lamb (115g)
- 1/2 tsp ground cumin (1g)
- 1/2 tsp smoked paprika (1g)
- 1/4 tsp salt (0.5g)
- 1/2 cup eggplant slices (75g)
- 1 tsp olive oil (5ml)
- 2 tbsp plain Greek yogurt (30g)
- 1 tsp fresh mint, chopped (2g)
- 1 tsp lemon juice (5ml)

Instructions:

1. Form lamb into 2 patties. Season with cumin, paprika, and salt.
2. Grill or pan-fry patties for 4–5 min per side.
3. Brush eggplant with olive oil and grill until tender.
4. Mix yogurt, mint, and lemon juice for sauce.
5. Serve patties with eggplant and yogurt.

Nutritional Facts (Per Serving): Calories: 488 | Carbohydrates: 6g | Protein: 24g | Fat: 20g | Sugar: 2g | Fiber: 2g | Sodium: 450mg

Glycemic Index: Lamb: 0 | Eggplant: 15 | Yogurt: 10

Paprika Pork Medallions with Warm Tomato-Olive Salsa

Prep: 10 minutes | **Cook:** 15 minutes | **Serves:** 1

Ingredients:

- 4 oz pork tenderloin, sliced into medallions (115g)
- 1/2 tsp paprika (1g)
- 1/2 tbsp olive oil (7ml)
- Salt and pepper to taste
- 1/2 cup cherry tomatoes, halved (75g)
- 1 tbsp pitted black olives, chopped (10g)
- 1 tsp red wine vinegar (5ml)
- 1/4 tsp oregano (0.5g)

Instructions:

1. Season pork with paprika, salt, and pepper. Sear in olive oil 3–4 min per side.
2. In a small pan, warm tomatoes, olives, oregano, and vinegar for 5 minutes.
3. Serve salsa over pork medallions.

Nutritional Facts (Per Serving): Calories: 492 | Carbohydrates: 8g | Protein: 25g | Fat: 19g | Sugar: 3g | Fiber: 2g | Sodium: 470mg

Glycemic Index: Pork: 0 | Tomato: 15 | Olives: 15

Chicken Thighs with Dijon-Caper Sauce

10 minutes | Cook: 20 minutes | Serves: 1

Ingredients:

- 1 boneless skinless chicken thigh (120g)
- 1/2 tbsp olive oil (7ml)
- 1 tsp Dijon mustard (5g)
- 1/2 tsp capers, chopped (2g)
- 1/4 cup low-sodium chicken broth (60ml)
- 1 cup spinach, fresh (30g)
- Salt and pepper to taste

Instructions:

1. Sear chicken thigh in olive oil, 5–6 min per side. Remove and keep warm.
2. In the same pan, add broth, mustard, capers, and deglaze for 3 min.
3. Return chicken to pan to coat in sauce.
4. Sauté spinach separately for 2–3 min with a drop of olive oil.
5. Serve together.

Nutritional Facts (Per Serving): Calories: 488 | Carbohydrates: 4g | Protein: 25g | Fat: 20g | Sugar: 1g | Fiber: 2g | Sodium: 470mg

Glycemic Index: Chicken: 0 | Spinach: 15 | Dijon: 35

Stuffed Cabbage Leaves with Beef and Herbs

Prep: 15 minutes | Cook: 25 minutes | Serves: 1

Ingredients:

- 2 large cabbage leaves (60g)
- 4 oz lean ground beef (115g)
- 1 tbsp onion, finely chopped (10g)
- 1 tbsp chopped parsley (5g)
- 1/2 clove garlic, minced (2g)
- 1 tsp olive oil (5ml)
- 1/4 cup low-sodium beef broth (60ml)
- Salt and pepper to taste

Instructions:

1. Blanch cabbage leaves 2 min in boiling water, then drain.
2. Mix beef, onion, garlic, parsley, salt, and pepper. Wrap into 2 cabbage rolls.
3. Sear rolls in olive oil 2–3 minutes. Add broth, cover, and simmer 15–20 min.
4. Serve with remaining pan juices.

Nutritional Facts (Per Serving): Calories: 475 | Carbohydrates: 7g | Protein: 24g | Fat: 19g | Sugar: 2g | Fiber: 3g | Sodium: 460mg

Glycemic Index: Beef: 0 | Cabbage: 15 | Onion: 10

Crispy Baked Pork Cutlets with Warm Fennel Slaw

Prep: 15 minutes | Cook: 25 minutes | Serves: 1

Ingredients:

- 4 oz pork loin, thinly sliced (115g)
- 1 tbsp almond flour (10g)
- 1/2 tsp garlic powder (0.5g)
- 1 tsp olive oil (5ml)
- Salt and pepper to taste
- 1/2 cup shredded fennel (50g)
- 1/4 cup shredded green cabbage (30g)
- 1 tsp lemon juice (5ml)

Instructions:

1. Preheat oven to 400°F (200°C).
2. Rub pork with garlic powder, salt, and pepper. Dredge lightly in almond flour.
3. Place on parchment-lined tray, spray or brush with oil. Bake 15–18 min.
4. Toss fennel and cabbage with lemon juice, warm in a pan 3–4 minutes.
5. Serve pork over slaw.

Nutritional Facts (Per Serving): Calories: 490 | Carbohydrates: 9g | Protein: 25g | Fat: 20g | Sugar: 2g | Fiber: 2g | Sodium: 450mg

Glycemic Index: Pork: 0 | Almond flour: 1 | Fennel: 15 | Cabbage: 15

Seared Duck Breast with Red Cabbage and Caraway

Prep: 10 minutes | Cook: 20 minutes | Serves: 1

Ingredients:

- 4 oz duck breast, skin on (115g)
- 1 cup shredded red cabbage (70g)
- 1/2 tsp caraway seeds (1g)
- 1 tsp apple cider vinegar (5ml)
- 1/2 tbsp olive oil (7ml)
- Salt and pepper to taste

Instructions:

1. Score duck skin, season with salt and pepper.
2. Sear skin-side down over medium heat for 5–6 min. Flip and cook 3–4 min. Rest 5 min before slicing.
3. Sauté red cabbage with olive oil and caraway seeds for 5–6 min. Add vinegar, cook 2 more min.
4. Serve sliced duck with warm cabbage.

Nutritional Facts (Per Serving): Calories: 495 | Carbohydrates: 7g | Protein: 24g | Fat: 20g | Sugar: 3g | Fiber: 2g | Sodium: 440mg

Glycemic Index: Duck: 0 | Cabbage: 15 | Vinegar: 5

Beef & Spinach Skillet with Cherry Tomatoes

Prep: 10 minutes | Cook: 15 minutes | Serves: 1

Ingredients:

- 4 oz lean beef strips (115g)
- 1 cup spinach, fresh (30g)
- 1/2 cup cherry tomatoes, halved (75g)
- 1 clove garlic, minced (3g)
- 1 tsp olive oil (5ml)
- Salt and pepper to taste

Instructions:

1. Heat olive oil in skillet. Add garlic and beef. Cook 5–6 min.
2. Add spinach and tomatoes. Sauté 3–4 min until wilted.
3. Season with salt and pepper. Serve hot.

Nutritional Facts (Per Serving): Calories: 485 | Carbohydrates: 6g | Protein: 24g | Fat: 20g | Sugar: 3g | Fiber: 2g | Sodium: 430mg

Glycemic Index: Beef: 0 | Spinach: 15 | Tomato: 30

Baked Chicken Drumsticks with Veggie Sauté

Prep: 10 minutes | Cook: 30 minutes | Serves: 1

Ingredients:

- 2 chicken drumsticks (150g)
- 1/2 medium zucchini, chopped (75g)
- 1/2 small tomato, chopped (50g)
- 1/2 tsp dried basil (0.5g)
- 1 tsp olive oil (5ml)
- Salt and pepper to taste

Instructions:

1. Preheat oven to 400°F (200°C). Season drumsticks with salt and pepper.
2. Bake for 30 minutes, turning halfway.
3. Meanwhile, sauté zucchini and tomato in olive oil with basil until soft.
4. Serve drumsticks with warm vegetable sauté.

Nutritional Facts (Per Serving): Calories: 480 | Carbohydrates: 8g | Protein: 24g | Fat: 19g | Sugar: 3g | Fiber: 2g | Sodium: 420mg

Glycemic Index: Chicken: 0 | Zucchini: 15 | Tomato: 30

CHAPTER 5: SNACKS AND DESSERTS: Healthy, Low-Carb Snacks to Keep You Satisfied

Cucumber Slices with Avocado and Hummus

Prep: 10 minutes | **Cook:** None | **Serves:** 2

Ingredients:

- 1 medium cucumber, sliced (200g)
- 1/2 avocado, mashed (75g)
- 2 tbsp hummus (30g)
- 1 tsp lemon juice (5ml)
- Pinch of salt and pepper

Instructions:

1. Arrange cucumber slices.
2. Mix avocado, hummus, lemon juice, salt, pepper.
3. Top each slice. Serve.

Nutritional Facts (Per Serving): Calories: 250 | Carbohydrates: 15g | Protein: 8g | Fat: 9g | Sugars: 3g | Fiber: 7g | Sodium: 250mg

Glycemic Index: Cucumber: Low (GI = 15) | Avocado: Negligible GI | Hummus: Low (GI = 15)

Stuffed Mini Bell Peppers with Cream Cheese and Herbs

Prep: 10 minutes | **Cook:** None | **Serves:** 2

Ingredients:

- 6 mini bell peppers (120g)
- 3 tbsp cream cheese, softened (45g)
- 1 tbsp fresh parsley, chopped (5g)
- 1 tsp lemon juice (5ml)
- Pinch of salt and pepper

Instructions:

1. Slice off the tops of the mini bell peppers and remove seeds.
2. Mix cream cheese with parsley, lemon juice, and a pinch of salt and pepper.
3. Stuff each bell pepper with the cream cheese mixture and serve.

Nutritional Facts (Per Serving): Calories: 250 | Carbohydrates: 12g | Protein: 9g | Fat: 9g | Sugars: 6g | Fiber: 4g | Sodium: 280mg

Glycemic Index: Bell peppers: Low (GI = 15) | Cream cheese: Low (GI = 15)

Bell Pepper Strips with Guacamole

Prep: 10 minutes | **Cook:** None | **Serves:** 2

Ingredients:

- 1 large bell pepper, sliced into strips (150g)
- 1/2 avocado, mashed (75g)
- 1 tbsp lime juice (15ml)
- 1 tbsp fresh cilantro, chopped (5g)
- Pinch of salt and pepper

Instructions:

1. Arrange bell pepper strips on a plate.
2. Mash avocado with lime juice and cilantro. Season with a pinch of salt and pepper.
3. Serve the bell pepper strips with the guacamole for dipping.

Nutritional Facts (Per Serving): Calories: 250 | Carbohydrates: 13g | Protein: 8g | Fat: 10g | Sugars: 5g | Fiber: 7g | Sodium: 220mg

Glycemic Index: Bell pepper: Low (GI = 15) | Avocado: Negligible GI | Lime juice: Negligible GI

Spinach and Ricotta Stuffed Mushrooms

Prep: 15 minutes | Cook: 15 minutes | Serves: 2

Ingredients:

- 6 large mushrooms (120g)
- 1/2 cup ricotta cheese (120g)
- 1/2 cup fresh spinach, chopped (30g)
- 1 tbsp grated Parmesan cheese (10g)
- 1 tsp olive oil (5ml)
- 1/4 tsp garlic powder (1g)
- Pinch of salt and pepper

Instructions:

1. Preheat the oven to 375°F (190°C).
2. Remove the stems from the mushrooms and set aside.
3. Mix ricotta, spinach, Parmesan, garlic powder, and a pinch of salt and pepper.
4. Stuff the mushroom caps with the mixture.
5. Drizzle olive oil over the stuffed mushrooms.
6. Bake for 12-15 minutes until mushrooms are tender.

Nutritional Facts (Per Serving): Calories: 250 | Carbohydrates: 10g | Protein: 9g | Fat: 10g | Sugars: 4g | Fiber: 3g | Sodium: 270mg

Glycemic Index: Mushrooms: Low (GI = 15) | Ricotta: Low (GI = 30) | Spinach: Negligible GI

Cauliflower in Cheese Batter

Prep: 10 minutes | Cook: 15 minutes | Serves: 2

Ingredients:

- 1/2 medium cauliflower, cut into florets (200g)
- 1/3 cup shredded cheddar cheese (40g)
- 1 large egg (50g)
- 2 tbsp almond flour (20g)
- 1 tbsp olive oil (15ml)
- 1/4 tsp paprika (1g)
- Pinch of salt and pepper

Instructions:

1. Preheat a skillet with olive oil over medium heat.
2. In a bowl, whisk the egg and mix in cheddar cheese, almond flour, paprika, salt, and pepper.
3. Dip cauliflower florets into the cheese batter.
4. Fry the cauliflower in the skillet until golden brown on all sides, about 5 minutes.

Nutritional Facts (Per Serving): Calories: 250 | Carbohydrates: 12g | Protein: 9g | Fat: 10g | Sugars: 3g | Fiber: 5g | Sodium: 280mg

Glycemic Index: Cauliflower: Low (GI = 15) | Cheese: Low (GI = 30) | Almond flour: Low (GI = 10)

Kale and Spinach Hummus with Almond Flour Crackers

Prep: 10 minutes | Cook: None | Serves: 2

Ingredients:

- 1/2 cup kale, chopped (30g)
- 1/2 cup spinach, chopped (30g)
- 1/4 cup hummus (60g)
- 1 tbsp lemon juice (15ml)
- 1 tsp olive oil (5ml)
- 1/4 tsp cumin (1g)
- Pinch of salt and pepper
- 6 almond flour crackers (30g)

Instructions:

1. Blend kale, spinach, hummus, lemon juice, olive oil, cumin, salt, and pepper until smooth.
2. Serve the hummus with almond flour crackers.

Nutritional Facts (Per Serving): Calories: 250 | Carbohydrates: 15g | Protein: 8g | Fat: 9g | Sugars: 3g | Fiber: 6g | Sodium: 250mg

Glycemic Index: Kale: Low (GI = 15) | Spinach: Negligible GI | Hummus: Low (GI = 15) | Almond flour crackers: Low (GI = 10)

Beetroot Hummus with Carrot and Zucchini Ribbons

Prep: 10 minutes | **Cook:** None | **Serves:** 2

Ingredients:

- 1/2 cup cooked beetroot, chopped (75g)
- 1/4 cup hummus (60g)
- 1 tbsp lemon juice (15ml)
- 1 tbsp olive oil (15ml)
- 1 medium carrot, peeled into ribbons (80g)
- 1 small zucchini, peeled into ribbons (100g)
- Pinch of salt and pepper

Instructions:

1. Blend beetroot, hummus, lemon juice, olive oil, and a pinch of salt and pepper until smooth.
2. Serve the beetroot hummus with carrot and zucchini ribbons for dipping.

Nutritional Facts (Per Serving): Calories: 250 | Carbohydrates: 18g | Protein: 9g | Fat: 10g | Sugars: 6g | Fiber: 5g | Sodium: 260mg

Glycemic Index: Beetroot: Medium (GI = 65) | Hummus: Low (GI = 15) | Carrot: Low (GI = 35) | Zucchini: Low (GI = 15)

Pumpkin Hummus with Cucumber

Prep: 10 minutes | **Cook:** None | **Serves:** 2

Ingredients:

- 1/2 cup canned pumpkin puree (120g)
- 1/4 cup hummus (60g)
- 1 tbsp olive oil (15ml)
- 1 tsp ground cumin (2g)
- 1 medium cucumber, sliced (200g)
- Pinch of salt and pepper

Instructions:

1. In a bowl, mix pumpkin puree, hummus, olive oil, cumin, and a pinch of salt and pepper until smooth.
2. Serve with cucumber slices for dipping.

Nutritional Facts (Per Serving): Calories: 250 | Carbohydrates: 20g | Protein: 8g | Fat: 9g | Sugars: 5g | Fiber: 6g | Sodium: 230mg

Glycemic Index: Pumpkin: Low (GI = 50) | Hummus: Low (GI = 15) | Cucumber: Low (GI = 15)

Olive and Sun-Dried Tomato Hummus with Zucchini

Prep: 10 minutes | **Cook:** None | **Serves:** 2

Ingredients:

- 1/4 cup hummus (60g)
- 1 tbsp chopped black olives (15g)
- 1 tbsp sun-dried tomatoes, chopped (10g)
- 1 tbsp olive oil (15ml)
- 1 small zucchini, sliced into rounds (100g)
- Pinch of salt and pepper

Instructions:

1. Stir together hummus, olives, sun-dried tomatoes, olive oil, and a pinch of salt and pepper.
2. Serve with zucchini slices for dipping.

Nutritional Facts (Per Serving): Calories: 250 | Carbohydrates: 16g | Protein: 8g | Fat: 10g | Sugars: 4g | Fiber: 5g | Sodium: 280mg

Glycemic Index: Hummus: Low (GI = 15) | Olives: Low (GI = 15) | Sun-dried tomatoes: Low (GI = 35) | Zucchini: Low (GI = 15)

Deviled Eggs with Smoked Salmon and Avocado Mousse

Prep: 15 minutes | Cook: None | Serves: 2

Ingredients:

- 4 large eggs, hard-boiled (200g)
- 1/2 avocado, mashed (75g)
- 2 oz smoked salmon, chopped (60g)
- 1 tbsp lemon juice (15ml)
- 1 tsp Dijon mustard (5g)
- Pinch of salt and pepper

Instructions:

1. Cut hard-boiled eggs in half and remove yolks.
2. In a bowl, mix mashed avocado, egg yolks, lemon juice, mustard, salt, and pepper.
3. Spoon the avocado mixture into the egg whites and top with smoked salmon.

Nutritional Facts (Per Serving): Calories: 250 | Carbohydrates: 6g | Protein: 10g | Fat: 9g | Sugars: 1g | Fiber: 3g | Sodium: 280mg

Glycemic Index: Eggs: Low (GI = Negligible) | Avocado: Negligible GI | Smoked salmon: Negligible GI

Cilantro Lime Hummus with Bell Pepper Strips

Prep: 10 minutes | Cook: None | Serves: 2

Ingredients:

- 1/4 cup hummus (60g)
- 1 tbsp fresh cilantro, chopped (5g)
- 1 tbsp lime juice (15ml)
- 1 small bell pepper, sliced (100g)
- 1 tsp olive oil (5ml)
- Pinch of salt and pepper

Instructions:

1. In a bowl, combine the hummus, chopped cilantro, and lime juice. Stir in the olive oil, salt, and pepper until smooth.
2. Slice the bell pepper into thin strips.
3. Serve the hummus with bell pepper strips for dipping.

Nutritional Facts (Per Serving): Calories: 250 | Carbohydrates: 20g | Protein: 8g | Fat: 9g | Sugars: 5g | Fiber: 6g | Sodium: 260mg

Glycemic Index: Hummus: Low (GI = 15) | Bell pepper: Low (GI = 15)

Low-Carb Whole Grain Pita with Basil Pesto and Feta

Prep: 10 minutes | Cook: None | Serves: 2

Ingredients:

- 1 small low-carb whole grain pita (40g)
- 2 tbsp basil pesto (30g)
- 2 tbsp crumbled feta cheese (30g)
- 1 tsp olive oil (5ml)
- Pinch of salt and pepper

Instructions:

1. Spread basil pesto over the pita.
2. Top with crumbled feta, drizzle with olive oil, and season with a pinch of salt and pepper.
3. Slice into quarters and serve.

Nutritional Facts (Per Serving): Calories: 250 | Carbohydrates: 16g | Protein: 9g | Fat: 9g | Sugars: 1g | Fiber: 4g | Sodium: 280mg

Glycemic Index: Whole grain pita: Low (GI = 50) | Pesto: Low (GI = 15) | Feta: Low (GI = 30)

Avocado Tuna Boats

Prep: 10 minutes | Cook: None | Serves: 2

Ingredients:

- 1 ripe avocado, halved and pitted (150g)
- 1 can tuna in water, drained (100g)
- 1 tbsp plain Greek yogurt (15g)
- 1 tsp lemon juice (5ml)
- 1 tsp chopped parsley (2g)
- Salt and black pepper to taste

Instructions:

1. In a bowl, mix tuna, yogurt, lemon juice, parsley, salt, and pepper.
2. Spoon the mixture into the avocado halves.
3. Serve immediately.

Nutritional Facts (Per Serving): Calories: 250 | Carbohydrates: 8g | Protein: 10g | Fat: 10g | Sugars: 1g | Fiber: 6g | Sodium: 270mg

Glycemic Index: Avocado: Negligible GI | Tuna: 0 | Yogurt: Low GI

Zucchini Chips with Parmesan Dust

Prep: 10 minutes | Cook: 15 minutes | Serves: 2

Ingredients:

- 1 medium zucchini, thinly sliced (150g)
- 2 tbsp grated Parmesan cheese (20g)
- 1 tsp olive oil (5ml)
- 1/4 tsp garlic powder (1g)
- Pinch of salt and pepper

Instructions:

1. Preheat oven to 400°F (200°C).
2. Toss zucchini slices with olive oil, garlic powder, salt, and pepper.
3. Place on parchment-lined baking tray. Sprinkle with Parmesan.
4. Bake for 12–15 minutes until crisp. Serve warm or cooled.

Nutritional Facts (Per Serving): Calories: 240 | Carbohydrates: 9g | Protein: 9g | Fat: 9g | Sugars: 3g | Fiber: 3g | Sodium: 260mg

Glycemic Index: Whole grain pita: Zucchini: 15 | Parmesan: 27

Celery Sticks with Almond Butter and Chia Seeds

Prep: 5 minutes | Cook: None | Serves: 2

Ingredients:

- 4 medium celery sticks (100g)
- 2 tbsp almond butter (30g)
- 1 tsp chia seeds (4g)

Instructions:

1. Spread almond butter into celery stalks.
2. Sprinkle chia seeds on top.
3. Serve immediately as a crunchy snack.

Nutritional Facts (Per Serving): Calories: 250 | Carbohydrates: 10g | Protein: 8g | Fat: 10g | Sugars: 2g | Fiber: 5g | Sodium: 240mg

Glycemic Index: Celery: 15 | Almond butter: 10 | Chia seeds: Low GI

Smoked Salmon Rolls with Cucumber and Cream Cheese

Prep: 10 minutes | **Cook:** None | **Serves:** 2

Ingredients:

- 4 slices smoked salmon (80g)
- 1/2 cucumber, cut into thin sticks (100g)
- 3 tbsp cream cheese (45g)
- 1 tsp lemon zest (1g)
- Pinch of black pepper

Instructions:

1. Spread cream cheese on each salmon slice.
2. Add cucumber sticks, sprinkle with lemon zest and pepper.
3. Roll up and serve.

Nutritional Facts (Per Serving): Calories: 240 | Carbohydrates: 6g | Protein: 10g | Fat: 10g | Sugars: 2g | Fiber: 2g | Sodium: 270mg

Glycemic Index: Salmon: 0 | Cucumber: 15 | Cream cheese: 15

Mini Eggplant Rounds with Herbed Goat Cheese

Prep: 10 minutes | **Cook:** 15 minutes | **Serves:** 2

Ingredients:

- 1 small eggplant, sliced into rounds (150g)
- 2 tbsp goat cheese (30g)
- 1/2 tsp dried oregano (1g)
- 1 tsp olive oil (5ml)
- Salt and pepper to taste

Instructions:

1. Preheat oven to 375°F (190°C).
2. Brush eggplant slices with olive oil and roast 12–15 min.
3. Top warm rounds with goat cheese, oregano, salt and pepper.
4. Serve warm or at room temperature.

Nutritional Facts (Per Serving): Calories: 240 | Carbohydrates: 9g | Protein: 9g | Fat: 9g | Sugars: 4g | Fiber: 4g | Sodium: 250mg

Glycemic Index: Eggplant: 15 | Goat cheese: 0

Hard-Boiled Eggs with Olive Tapenade

Prep: 5 minutes | **Cook:** 10 minutes | **Serves:** 2

Ingredients:

- 4 large eggs, hard-boiled (200g)
- 2 tbsp olive tapenade (30g)
- Pinch of black pepper

Instructions:

1. Peel and halve hard-boiled eggs.
2. Top each half with a small spoonful of olive tapenade.
3. Sprinkle with black pepper and serve.

Nutritional Facts (Per Serving): Calories: 245 | Carbohydrates: 4g | Protein: 10g | Fat: 9g | Sugars: 1g | Fiber: 2g | Sodium: 260mg

Glycemic Index: Eggs: 0 | Olives: 15

Stuffed Cherry Tomatoes with Avocado and Tuna

Prep: 10 minutes | **Cook:** None | **Serves:** 2

Ingredients:

- 10 cherry tomatoes, tops removed and hollowed (150g)
- 1/2 avocado, mashed (75g)
- 2 tbsp canned tuna, drained (30g)
- 1/2 tsp lemon juice (2.5ml)
- Pinch of salt and pepper

Instructions:

1. Mix mashed avocado with tuna, lemon juice, salt, and pepper.
2. Fill each tomato with the mixture.
3. Serve immediately or chill.

Nutritional Facts (Per Serving): Calories: 250 | Carbohydrates: 9g | Protein: 9g | Fat: 10g | Sugars: 4g | Fiber: 4g | Sodium: 240mg

Glycemic Index: Tomato: 30 | Avocado: 0 | Tuna: 0

Cottage Cheese with Walnuts and Cinnamon

Prep: 5 minutes | **Cook:** None | **Serves:** 2

Ingredients:

- 1/2 cup cottage cheese, low-fat (120g)
- 2 tbsp chopped walnuts (20g)
- 1/4 tsp ground cinnamon (0.5g)
- Optional: 1–2 drops monk fruit sweetener

Instructions:

1. In a bowl, mix cottage cheese with cinnamon and sweetener (if using).
2. Top with chopped walnuts and serve.

Nutritional Facts (Per Serving): Calories: 245 | Carbohydrates: 8g | Protein: 10g | Fat: 10g | Sugars: 2g | Fiber: 2g | Sodium: 220mg

Glycemic Index: Cottage cheese: 30 | Walnuts: 15 | Cinnamon: 0

Radish Slices with Herbed Cream Cheese

Prep: 5 minutes | **Cook:** None | **Serves:** 2

Ingredients:

- 1 cup radishes, thinly sliced (100g)
- 2 tbsp cream cheese (30g)
- 1 tsp chopped fresh dill (2g)
- Pinch of salt and pepper

Instructions:

1. Mix cream cheese with dill, salt, and pepper.
2. Spread a little on each radish slice.
3. Serve as bite-sized canapés.

Nutritional Facts (Per Serving): Calories: 240 | Carbohydrates: 7g | Protein: 8g | Fat: 9g | Sugars: 2g | Fiber: 3g | Sodium: 210mg

Glycemic Index: Radish: 15 | Cream cheese: 15

High-Protein Options to Curb Cravings

Cottage Cheese with Sliced Tomatoes and Cucumber

Prep: 5 minutes | **Cook:** None | **Serves:** 2

Ingredients:

- 1/2 cup cottage cheese (120g)
- 1 medium tomato, sliced (120g)
- 1/2 cucumber, sliced (100g)
- 1 tsp olive oil (5ml)
- Pinch of salt and pepper

Instructions:

1. Arrange sliced tomatoes and cucumber on a plate.
2. Add cottage cheese on the side.
3. Drizzle olive oil over the vegetables and season with salt and pepper.

Nutritional Facts (Per Serving): Calories: 250 | Carbohydrates: 12g | Protein: 10g | Fat: 9g | Sugars: 7g | Fiber: 2g | Sodium: 260mg

Glycemic Index: Cottage cheese: Low (GI = 30) | Tomato: Low (GI = 15) | Cucumber: Low (GI = 15)

Turkey and Cheese Skewers with Olives

Prep: 10 minutes | **Cook:** None | **Serves:** 2

Ingredients:

- 3 oz turkey breast, cubed (85g)
- 2 oz cheddar cheese, cubed (60g)
- 8 black olives (40g)
- 1 tbsp olive oil (15ml)
- 1 tsp dried oregano (1g)

Instructions:

1. Thread turkey, cheese, and olives onto skewers.
2. Drizzle with olive oil and sprinkle with dried oregano.

Nutritional Facts (Per Serving): Calories: 250 | Carbohydrates: 3g | Protein: 10g | Fat: 10g | Sugars: 0g | Fiber: 1g | Sodium: 280mg

Glycemic Index: Turkey: Negligible GI | Cheese: Low (GI = 30) | Olives: Low (GI = 15)

Sliced Chicken Breast with Guacamole and Veggies

Prep: 10 minutes | **Cook:** 15 minutes | **Serves:** 2

Ingredients:

- 4 oz cooked chicken breast, sliced (120g)
- 1/4 cup guacamole (60g)
- 1 small bell pepper, sliced (100g)
- 1/2 cucumber, sliced (100g)
- Pinch of salt and pepper

Instructions:

1. Arrange sliced chicken breast on a plate.
2. Serve with guacamole, bell pepper, and cucumber slices on the side.
3. Season with salt and pepper.

Nutritional Facts (Per Serving): Calories: 250 | Carbohydrates: 12g | Protein: 9g | Fat: 10g | Sugars: 4g | Fiber: 5g | Sodium: 270mg

Glycemic Index: Chicken: Negligible GI | Guacamole: Low (GI = 15) | Bell pepper: Low (GI = 15) | Cucumber: Low (GI = 15)

Tuna-Stuffed Avocados with Olive Oil and Lemon

Prep: 10 minutes | Cook: None | Serves: 2

Ingredients:

- 1 medium avocado, halved (150g)
- 1/2 cup canned tuna, drained (120g)
- 1 tbsp olive oil (15ml)
- 1 tbsp lemon juice (15ml)
- Pinch of salt and pepper

Instructions:

1. Scoop out a little of the avocado flesh to make a larger cavity.
2. Mix tuna with olive oil, lemon juice, salt, and pepper.
3. Stuff the tuna mixture into the avocado halves.

Nutritional Facts (Per Serving): Calories: 250 | Carbohydrates: 9g | Protein: 10g | Fat: 10g | Sugars: 1g | Fiber: 5g | Sodium: 270mg

Glycemic Index: Avocado: Negligible GI | Tuna: Negligible GI | Lemon juice: Negligible GI

Turkey and Avocado Lettuce Wraps

Prep: 10 minutes | Cook: None | Serves: 2

Ingredients:

- 3 oz sliced turkey breast (85g)
- 1/2 avocado, sliced (75g)
- 4 large lettuce leaves (60g)
- 1 tbsp lime juice (15ml)
- 1 tbsp olive oil (15ml)
- Pinch of salt and pepper

Instructions:

1. Lay out the lettuce leaves and fill with turkey slices and avocado.
2. Drizzle with lime juice and olive oil, and season with salt and pepper.
3. Wrap and serve.

Nutritional Facts (Per Serving): Calories: 250 | Carbohydrates: 6g | Protein: 9g | Fat: 10g | Sugars: 1g | Fiber: 3g | Sodium: 260mg

Glycemic Index: Turkey: Negligible GI | Avocado: Negligible GI | Lettuce: Negligible GI

Hard-Boiled Eggs with Cottage Cheese and Spinach

Prep: 5 minutes | Cook: 10 minutes | Serves: 2

Ingredients:

- 2 large hard-boiled eggs (100g)
- 1/2 cup cottage cheese (120g)
- 1/2 cup fresh spinach, chopped (30g)
- 1 tsp olive oil (5ml)
- Pinch of salt and pepper

Instructions:

1. Slice hard-boiled eggs and arrange on a plate.
2. Top with cottage cheese and chopped spinach.
3. Drizzle with olive oil and season with salt and pepper.

Nutritional Facts (Per Serving): Calories: 250 | Carbohydrates: 8g | Protein: 10g | Fat: 9g | Sugars: 2g | Fiber: 2g | Sodium: 250mg

Glycemic Index: Eggs: Negligible GI | Cottage cheese: Low (GI = 30) | Spinach: Negligible GI

Tuna Salad Lettuce Cups with Olive Oil

Prep: 10 minutes | **Cook:** None | **Serves:** 2

Ingredients:

- 1/2 cup canned tuna, drained (120g)
- 1 tbsp olive oil (15ml)
- 1 tbsp lemon juice (15ml)
- 1 tbsp chopped parsley (5g)
- 4 large lettuce leaves (60g)
- Pinch of salt and pepper

Instructions:

1. In a bowl, mix tuna, olive oil, lemon juice, parsley, salt, and pepper.
2 Spoon the tuna mixture into the lettuce leaves and serve.

Nutritional Facts (Per Serving): Calories: 250 | Carbohydrates: 3g | Protein: 10g | Fat: 10g | Sugars: 0g | Fiber: 2g | Sodium: 270mg

Glycemic Index: Tuna: Negligible GI | Lettuce: Low (GI = 15) | Lemon juice: Negligible GI

Chicken Salad with Avocado and Chia Seeds

Prep: 10 minutes | **Cook:** None | **Serves:** 2

Ingredients:

- 3 oz cooked chicken breast, diced (85g)
- 1/2 avocado, diced (75g)
- 1 tbsp chia seeds (10g)
- 1 tbsp olive oil (15ml)
- 1 tbsp lime juice (15ml)
- Pinch of salt and pepper

Instructions:

1. In a bowl, combine diced chicken, avocado, chia seeds, olive oil, lime juice, salt, and pepper.
2. Mix well and serve.

Nutritional Facts (Per Serving): Calories: 250 | Carbohydrates: 8g | Protein: 10g | Fat: 10g | Sugars: 0g | Fiber: 5g | Sodium: 260mg

Glycemic Index: Chicken: Negligible GI | Avocado: Negligible GI | Chia seeds: Low (GI = 1)

Spinach Egg Bites with Cottage Cheese

Prep: 10 minutes | **Cook:** 15 minutes | **Serves:** 2

Ingredients:

- 2 large eggs (100g)
- 1/2 cup cottage cheese (120g)
- 1 cup fresh spinach, chopped (30g)
- 1 tbsp chopped parsley (5g)
- Salt and pepper to taste

Instructions:

1. Preheat oven to 350°F (175°C).
2. Mix all ingredients in a bowl.
3. Pour into greased muffin cups and bake for 15 minutes until firm.
4. Cool slightly and serve.

Nutritional Facts (Per Serving): Calories: 245 | Carbohydrates: 5g | Protein: 10g | Fat: 10g | Sugars: 2g | Fiber: 1g | Sodium: 260mg

Glycemic Index: Eggs: 0 | Cottage cheese: 30 | Spinach: 15

Chicken & Avocado Pita Wedges

Prep: 10 minutes | Cook: None | Serves: 2

Ingredients:

- 3 oz cooked chicken breast, diced (85g)
- 1/2 avocado, mashed (75g)
- 1 small low-carb pita, sliced into quarters (40g)
- 1 tsp lemon juice (5ml)
- Pinch of salt and pepper

Instructions:

1. Mix avocado with lemon juice, salt, and pepper.
2. Spread onto pita slices, top with chicken.
3. Serve as open-faced mini wedges.

Nutritional Facts (Per Serving): Calories: 250 | Carbohydrates: 12g | Protein: 10g | Fat: 10g | Sugars: 1g | Fiber: 4g | Sodium: 270mg

Glycemic Index: Pita (low-carb): ~45 | Avocado: 0 | Chicken: 0

Ricotta-Stuffed Sweet Mini Peppers

Prep: 10 minutes | Cook: None | Serves: 2

Ingredients:

- 6 mini sweet peppers, halved and seeded (120g)
- 1/2 cup low-fat ricotta cheese (120g)
- 1 tsp olive oil (5ml)
- 1/2 tsp dried basil (1g)
- Salt and pepper to taste

Instructions:

1. Mix ricotta, olive oil, basil, salt, and pepper.
2. Fill pepper halves with mixture.
3. Serve chilled or room temp.

Nutritional Facts (Per Serving): Calories: 240 | Carbohydrates: 8g | Protein: 10g | Fat: 9g | Sugars: 4g | Fiber: 2g | Sodium: 250mg

Glycemic Index: Peppers: 15 | Ricotta: 30 | Olive oil: 0

Turkey and Cucumber Roll-Ups with Mustard Dip

Prep: 10 minutes | Cook: None | Serves: 2

Ingredients:

- 3 oz turkey breast, thinly sliced (85g)
- 1/2 cucumber, sliced into sticks (100g)
- 1 tbsp plain Greek yogurt (15g)
- 1/2 tsp Dijon mustard (2g)
- Salt and pepper to taste

Instructions:

1. Roll cucumber sticks inside turkey slices.
2. Mix yogurt and mustard for dip.
3. Serve turkey rolls with dip on the side.

Nutritional Facts (Per Serving): Calories: 240 | Carbs: 5g | Protein: 10g | Fat: 9g | Sugar: 1g | Fiber: 1g | Sodium: 250mg

Glycemic Index: Turkey: 0 | Cucumber: 15 | Yogurt: ~30

Tofu Salad with Greens and Lemon-Oil Dressing

Prep: 10 minutes | Cook: None | Serves: 2

Ingredients:

- 1/2 cup firm tofu, cubed (100g)
- 1 cup mixed leafy greens (30g)
- 1 tbsp olive oil (15ml)
- 1 tbsp lemon juice (15ml)
- Salt and pepper to taste

Instructions:

1. Toss tofu and greens with olive oil, lemon juice, salt, and pepper.
2. Serve fresh.

Nutritional Facts (Per Serving): Calories: 245 | Carbs: 6g | Protein: 10g | Fat: 10g | Sugar: 1g | Fiber: 2g | Sodium: 240mg

Glycemic Index: Tofu: ~15 | Greens: ~10 | Olive oil: 0

Egg and Veggie Cups with Bell Pepper and Onion

Prep: 10 minutes | Cook: 15 minutes | Serves: 2

Ingredients:

- 2 large eggs (100g)
- 1/4 cup diced red bell pepper (50g)
- 1/4 cup diced onion (50g)
- 1 tsp olive oil (5ml)
- Salt and pepper to taste

Instructions:

1. Preheat oven to 350°F (175°C).
2. Sauté bell pepper and onion in olive oil for 3–4 minutes.
3. Mix with beaten eggs, pour into muffin cups, and bake for 12–15 minutes.
4. Serve warm.

Nutritional Facts (Per Serving): Calories: 240 | Carbs: 7g | Protein: 10g | Fat: 10g | Sugar: 3g | Fiber: 1g | Sodium: 230mg

Glycemic Index: Eggs: 0 | Bell Pepper: 15 | Onion: 10

Avocado & Egg Mash on Zucchini Rounds

Prep: 10 minutes | Cook: None | Serves: 2

Ingredients:

- 1 boiled egg, chopped (50g)
- 1/2 avocado, mashed (75g)
- 1 small zucchini, sliced into rounds (100g)
- 1 tsp lemon juice (5ml)
- Pinch of salt and pepper

Instructions:

1. Mix chopped egg, avocado, lemon juice, salt, and pepper.
2. Spoon onto raw zucchini rounds.
3. Serve fresh as finger snacks.

Nutritional Facts (Per Serving): Calories: 245 | Carbs: 7g | Protein: 9g | Fat: 10g | Sugar: 2g | Fiber: 4g | Sodium: 240mg

Glycemic Index: Avocado: 0 | Egg: 0 | Zucchini: 15

Low-Sugar Dessert Recipes That Don't Spike Blood Sugar

Almond Flour Brownies with Dark Chocolate

Prep: 10 minutes | **Cook:** 20 minutes | **Serves:** 4

Ingredients:

- 1/2 cup almond flour (50g)
- 2 oz dark chocolate, melted (60g)
- 2 tbsp low carb sweetener (24g)
- 1 large egg (50g)
- 2 tbsp unsweetened cocoa powder (15g)
- 1 tbsp olive oil (15ml)
- 1/2 tsp vanilla extract (2.5ml)
- Pinch of salt

Instructions:

1. Preheat oven to 350°F (180°C) and grease a small baking pan.
2. In a bowl, mix almond flour, melted dark chocolate, egg, sweetener, cocoa powder, olive oil, vanilla extract, and salt until smooth.
3. Pour the batter into the baking pan and bake for 15-20 minutes. Let cool before slicing.

Nutritional Facts (Per Serving): Calories: 250 | Carbohydrates: 10g | Protein: 9g | Fat: 10g | Sugars: 3g | Fiber: 5g | Sodium: 200mg

Glycemic Index: Almond flour: Low (GI = 10) | Dark chocolate: Low (GI = 25)

Coconut Chia Pudding with Berries

Prep: 5 minutes | **Cook:** None | **Serves:** 2

Ingredients:

- 1/2 cup coconut milk (120ml)
- 2 tbsp chia seeds (30g)
- 1 tbsp low carb sweetener (12g)
- 1/4 cup mixed berries (40g)
- 1/2 tsp vanilla extract (2.5ml)

Instructions:

1. In a bowl, whisk coconut milk, chia seeds, sweetener, and vanilla extract.
2. Refrigerate for 2 hours until thickened.
3. Top with mixed berries and serve.

Nutritional Facts (Per Serving): Calories: 250 | Carbohydrates: 12g | Protein: 8g | Fat: 10g | Sugars: 4g | Fiber: 6g | Sodium: 100mg

Glycemic Index: Chia seeds: Low (GI = 1) | Berries: Low (GI = 25) | Coconut milk: Low (GI = 40)

Sugar-Free Lemon Cheesecake Bites

Prep: 10 minutes | **Cook:** 15 minutes | **Serves:** 4

Ingredients:

- 4 oz cream cheese, softened (120g)
- 1 tbsp low carb sweetener (12g)
- 1 tbsp lemon juice (15ml)
- 1 large egg (50g)
- 1/2 tsp lemon zest (1g)

Instructions:

1. Preheat oven to 350°F (180°C) and grease a muffin tin.
2. In a bowl, mix cream cheese, sweetener, lemon juice, lemon zest, and egg until smooth.
3. Pour the mixture into the muffin tin and bake for 12-15 minutes. Let cool before serving.

Nutritional Facts (Per Serving): Calories: 250 | Carbohydrates: 5g | Protein: 9g | Fat: 10g | Sugars: 2g | Fiber: 1g | Sodium: 220mg

Glycemic Index: Cream cheese: Low (GI = 30) | Lemon juice: Negligible GI

Low-Sugar Chocolate Avocado Mousse

Prep: 10 minutes | Cook: None | Serves: 2

Ingredients:

- 1 ripe avocado (150g)
- 2 tbsp unsweetened cocoa powder (15g)
- 2 tbsp low carb sweetener (24g)
- 1/4 cup almond milk (60ml)
- 1 tsp vanilla extract (5ml)

Instructions:

1. Blend avocado, cocoa powder, low carb sweetener, almond milk, and vanilla extract until smooth.
2. Serve chilled in small bowls or cups.

Nutritional Facts (Per Serving): Calories: 250 | Carbohydrates: 12g | Protein: 9g | Fat: 10g | Sugars: 2g | Fiber: 6g | Sodium: 100mg

Glycemic Index: Avocado: Negligible GI | Cocoa: Low (GI = 20) | Almond milk: Low (GI = 30)

Keto-Friendly Berry Cheesecake Bars

Prep: 15 minutes | Cook: 25 minutes | Serves: 4

Ingredients:

- 1/2 cup almond flour (50g)
- 2 tbsp low carb sweetener (24g)
- 1/4 cup butter, melted (60ml)
- 4 oz cream cheese, softened (120g)
- 1/4 cup mixed berries (50g)
- 1 large egg (50g)
- 1/2 tsp vanilla extract (2.5ml)

Instructions:

1. Preheat oven to 350°F (180°C). Mix almond flour, 1 tbsp sweetener, and melted butter for the crust. Press into a small baking dish and bake for 10 minutes.
2. In a bowl, mix cream cheese, egg, remaining sweetener, and vanilla extract until smooth. Spread over the crust and top with berries.
3. Bake for another 15 minutes, then let cool before cutting into bars.

Nutritional Facts (Per Serving): Calories: 250 | Carbohydrates: 10g | Protein: 9g | Fat: 10g | Sugars: 3g | Fiber: 4g | Sodium: 220mg

Glycemic Index: Almond flour: Low (GI = 10) | Cream cheese: Low (GI = 30) | Berries: Low (GI = 25)

Sugar-Free Almond Butter Cups

Prep: 10 minutes | Cook: 5 minutes | Serves: 4

Ingredients:

- 1/4 cup almond butter (60g)
- 1/4 cup dark chocolate, melted (60g)
- 1 tbsp coconut oil (15ml)
- 1 tbsp low carb sweetener (12g)
- 1/2 tsp vanilla extract (2.5ml)

Instructions:

1. Mix almond butter with 1/2 tbsp coconut oil and vanilla extract.
2. Melt dark chocolate with remaining coconut oil and low carb sweetener.
3. Pour half the chocolate mixture into silicone muffin cups, spoon almond butter mixture on top, and cover with the remaining chocolate.
4. Freeze for 10-15 minutes until set.

Nutritional Facts (Per Serving): Calories: 250 | Carbohydrates: 8g | Protein: 9g | Fat: 10g | Sugars: 3g | Fiber: 4g | Sodium: 200mg

Glycemic Index: Almond butter: Low (GI = 15) | Dark chocolate: Low (GI = 25)

Keto Pumpkin Pie Bites with Coconut Cream

Prep: 15 minutes | Cook: 10 minutes | Serves: 4

Ingredients:

- 1/2 cup pumpkin puree (120g)
- 1/4 cup almond flour (30g)
- 1 tbsp low carb sweetener (12g)
- 1 large egg (50g)
- 1 tsp pumpkin pie spice (2g)
- 1/2 tsp vanilla extract (2.5ml)
- 1/4 cup coconut cream (60ml)

Instructions:

1. Preheat oven to 350°F (180°C).
2. Mix pumpkin puree, almond flour, sweetener, egg, pumpkin pie spice, and vanilla extract.
3. Spoon the mixture into mini muffin tins and bake for 10 minutes.
4. Serve with a dollop of coconut cream on top.

Nutritional Facts (Per Serving): Calories: 250 | Carbohydrates: 10g | Protein: 8g | Fat: 10g | Sugars: 3g | Fiber: 4g | Sodium: 200mg

Glycemic Index: Pumpkin: Low (GI = 50) | Almond flour: Low (GI = 10) | Coconut cream: Low (GI = 40)

Cinnamon Almond Butter Cookies

Prep: 10 minutes | Cook: 12 minutes | Serves: 4

Ingredients:

- 1/2 cup almond butter (120g)
- 1 large egg (50g)
- 2 tbsp low carb sweetener (24g)
- 1 tsp ground cinnamon (2g)
- 1/2 tsp baking powder (2g)
- 1/2 tsp vanilla extract (2.5ml)

Instructions:

1. Preheat oven to 350°F (180°C).
2. Mix almond butter, egg, sweetener, cinnamon, baking powder, and vanilla extract until smooth.
3. Drop spoonfuls of dough onto a baking sheet and flatten slightly.
4. Bake for 10-12 minutes, then let cool before serving.

Nutritional Facts (Per Serving): Calories: 250 | Carbohydrates: 8g | Protein: 9g | Fat: 10g | Sugars: 2g | Fiber: 4g | Sodium: 200mg

Glycemic Index: Almond butter: Low (GI = 15) | Cinnamon: Negligible GI

Keto Lemon Bars with Coconut Crust

Prep: 15 minutes | Cook: 20 minutes | Serves: 4

Ingredients:

- 1/2 cup almond flour (50g)
- 1/4 cup shredded coconut (30g)
- 2 tbsp low carb sweetener (24g)
- 1/4 cup butter, melted (60ml)
- 1 large egg (50g)
- 2 tbsp lemon juice (30ml)
- 1 tsp lemon zest (2g)

Instructions:

1. Preheat oven to 350°F (180°C). Mix almond flour, shredded coconut, 1 tbsp sweetener, and melted butter to form the crust. Press into a small baking dish and bake for 10 minutes.
2. In a bowl, whisk egg, lemon juice, remaining sweetener, and lemon zest. Pour over the crust.
3. Bake for an additional 10 minutes. Let cool and slice into bars.

Nutritional Facts (Per Serving): Calories: 250 | Carbohydrates: 10g | Protein: 8g | Fat: 10g | Sugars: 2g | Fiber: 5g | Sodium: 220mg

Glycemic Index: Almond flour: Low (GI = 10) | Coconut: Low (GI = 45) | Lemon juice: Negligible GI

Lemon Poppy Seed Muffins with Almond Flour

Prep: 10 minutes | **Cook:** 20 minutes | **Serves:** 4

Ingredients:

- 1 cup almond flour (100g)
- 2 large eggs (100g)
- 2 tbsp low carb sweetener (24g)
- 1 tbsp poppy seeds (10g)
- 2 tbsp lemon juice (30ml)
- 1 tsp lemon zest (2g)
- 1/2 tsp baking powder (2g)

Instructions:

1. Preheat oven to 350°F (180°C).
2. In a bowl, mix almond flour, sweetener, poppy seeds, lemon juice, lemon zest, eggs, and baking powder until smooth.
3. Pour the batter into muffin tins and bake for 18-20 minutes.
4. Let cool before serving.

Nutritional Facts (Per Serving): Calories: 250 | Carbohydrates: 8g | Protein: 9g | Fat: 10g | Sugars: 2g | Fiber: 4g | Sodium: 200mg

Glycemic Index: Almond flour: Low (GI = 10) | Poppy seeds: Low (GI = 15) | Lemon juice: Negligible GI

Strawberry and Coconut Cream Chia Parfait

Prep: 10 minutes | **Cook:** None | **Serves:** 2

Ingredients:

- 1/2 cup coconut milk (120ml)
- 2 tbsp chia seeds (30g)
- 1 tbsp low carb sweetener (12g)
- 1/4 cup strawberries, sliced (40g)
- 1 tbsp shredded coconut (7g)

Instructions:

1. In a bowl, whisk coconut milk, chia seeds, and sweetener. Refrigerate for 2 hours until thickened.
2. Layer chia pudding with sliced strawberries in glasses.
3. Top with shredded coconut and serve.

Nutritional Facts (Per Serving): Calories: 250 | Carbohydrates: 12g | Protein: 8g | Fat: 10g | Sugars: 4g | Fiber: 6g | Sodium: 100mg

Glycemic Index: Chia seeds: Low (GI = 1) | Strawberries: Low (GI = 25) | Coconut milk: Low (GI = 40)

Keto Chocolate Lava Cake with Dark Chocolate Filling

Prep: 10 minutes | **Cook:** 12 minutes | **Serves:** 2

Ingredients:

- 2 oz dark chocolate (60g)
- 2 tbsp butter (30g)
- 1 large egg (50g)
- 1 tbsp almond flour (10g)
- 1 tbsp low carb sweetener (12g)
- 1/2 tsp vanilla extract (2.5ml)

Instructions:

1. Preheat oven to 400°F (200°C) and grease two small ramekins.
2. Melt dark chocolate and butter together.
3. In a separate bowl, whisk egg, sweetener, almond flour, and vanilla extract.
4. Combine the chocolate mixture with the egg mixture.
5. Pour into the ramekins and bake for 10-12 minutes until the edges are set but the center is still soft.
6. Let cool slightly before serving.

Nutritional Facts (Per Serving): Calories: 250 | Carbohydrates: 12g | Protein: 9g | Fat: 10g | Sugars: 3g | Fiber: 4g | Sodium: 150mg

Glycemic Index: Dark chocolate: Low (GI = 25) | Almond flour: Low (GI = 10)

Almond Flour Snickerdoodle Cookies

Prep: 10 minutes | Cook: 12 minutes | Serves: 4

Ingredients:

- 1 cup almond flour (100g)
- 1 large egg (50g)
- 2 tbsp low carb sweetener (24g)
- 1/4 tsp baking soda (1g)
- 1/2 tsp cinnamon (1g)
- 1/2 tsp vanilla extract (2.5ml)
- 1 tbsp melted butter (15g)

Instructions:

1. Preheat oven to 350°F (180°C) and line a baking sheet with parchment paper.
2. In a bowl, mix almond flour, sweetener, baking soda, and cinnamon.
3. Add egg, melted butter, and vanilla extract. Stir until combined.
4. Roll dough into small balls, flatten slightly, and place on the baking sheet.
5. Bake for 10-12 minutes, until golden brown. Let cool before serving.

Nutritional Facts (Per Serving): Calories: 250 | Carbohydrates: 8g | Protein: 9g | Fat: 10g | Sugars: 2g | Fiber: 3g | Sodium: 220mg

Glycemic Index: Almond flour: Low (GI = 10) | Cinnamon: Negligible GI

Coconut Matcha Energy Balls

Prep: 10 minutes | Cook: None | Serves: 4

Ingredients:

- 1/2 cup shredded coconut (40g)
- 2 tbsp almond flour (20g)
- 1 tbsp matcha powder (5g)
- 2 tbsp low carb sweetener (24g)
- 2 tbsp coconut oil, melted (30ml)
- 1 tsp vanilla extract (5ml)

Instructions:

1. In a bowl, mix shredded coconut, almond flour, matcha powder, sweetener, and vanilla extract.
2. Add melted coconut oil and stir until the mixture holds together.
3. Roll into small balls and refrigerate for 30 minutes before serving.

Nutritional Facts (Per Serving): Calories: 250 | Carbohydrates: 10g | Protein: 8g | Fat: 10g | Sugars: 2g | Fiber: 5g | Sodium: 200mg

Glycemic Index: Shredded coconut: Low (GI = 45) | Matcha: Low (GI = 1)

Sugar-Free Raspberry Mousse with Whipped Coconut Cream

Prep: 10 minutes | Cook: None | Serves: 2

Ingredients:

- 1/2 cup raspberries (60g)
- 1/4 cup coconut cream (60ml)
- 2 tbsp low carb sweetener (24g)
- 1/2 tsp vanilla extract (2.5ml)

Instructions:

1. Blend raspberries and sweetener until smooth.
2. In a separate bowl, whip coconut cream and vanilla extract until fluffy.
3. Gently fold the raspberry mixture into the whipped coconut cream.
4. Serve chilled.

Nutritional Facts (Per Serving): Calories: 250 | Carbohydrates: 10g | Protein: 8g | Fat: 10g | Sugars: 3g | Fiber: 5g | Sodium: 100mg

Glycemic Index: Raspberries: Low (GI = 25) | Coconut cream: Low (GI = 40)

Banana Nut Oat Bars with Almond Butter

Prep: 10 minutes | **Cook:** 20 minutes | **Serves:** 4

Ingredients:

- 1 ripe banana, mashed (100g)
- 1/2 cup rolled oats (50g)
- 2 tbsp almond butter (30g)
- 1 tbsp low carb sweetener (12g)
- 1/4 cup chopped walnuts (30g)
- 1 large egg (50g)
- 1/2 tsp vanilla extract (2.5ml)

Instructions:

1. Preheat oven to 350°F (180°C).
2. In a bowl, mix mashed banana, oats, almond butter, sweetener, walnuts, egg, and vanilla extract.
3. Pour the mixture into a baking pan and press down evenly.
4. Bake for 18-20 minutes until golden. Let cool before cutting into bars.

Nutritional Facts (Per Serving): Calories: 250 | Carbohydrates: 20g | Protein: 9g | Fat: 10g | Sugars: 5g | Fiber: 4g | Sodium: 220mg

Glycemic Index: Banana: Medium (GI = 51) | Oats: Low (GI = 55) | Almond butter: Low (GI = 15)

Blueberry Almond Mug Cake

Prep: 5 minutes | **Cook:** 2 minutes | **Serves:** 2

Ingredients:

- 1/2 cup almond flour (50g)
- 1 tbsp monk fruit sweetener (12g)
- 1 egg (50g)
- 2 tbsp unsweetened almond milk (30ml)
- 1/4 tsp baking powder (1g)
- 1/4 tsp vanilla extract (1.25ml)
- 2 tbsp fresh blueberries (30g)

Instructions:

1. In a bowl, whisk egg, almond flour, sweetener, almond milk, baking powder, and vanilla extract until smooth.
2. Fold in blueberries.
3. Pour into a microwave-safe mug and microwave for 90–120 seconds.
4. Let cool slightly and serve.

Nutritional Facts (Per Serving): Calories: 250 | Carbs: 10g | Protein: 9g | Fat: 10g | Sugar: 3g | Fiber: 4g | Sodium: 220mg

Glycemic Index: Almond flour: Low (GI = 10) | Blueberries: Low (GI = 25)

Cacao Coconut Bites with Allulose

Prep: 10 minutes | **Cook:** None | **Serves:** 2

Ingredients:

- 1/4 cup shredded coconut (30g)
- 1 tbsp unsweetened cocoa powder (8g)
- 1 tbsp allulose (12g)
- 2 tbsp almond flour (20g)
- 1 tbsp coconut oil, melted (15ml)
- 1/4 tsp vanilla extract (1.25ml)

Instructions:

1. Mix all ingredients in a bowl until well combined.
2. Form into small balls using hands or a scoop.
3. Chill in the refrigerator for 30 minutes before serving.

Nutritional Facts (Per Serving): Calories: 250 | Carbs: 9g | Protein: 8g | Fat: 10g | Sugar: 2g | Fiber: 5g | Sodium: 200mg

Glycemic Index: Coconut: Low (GI = 45) | Cocoa powder: Low (GI = 20)

Mini Lemon Ricotta Cups with Coconut Crust

Prep: 10 minutes | Cook: 15 minutes | Serves: 2

Ingredients:

- 1/4 cup ricotta cheese (60g)
- 1 tbsp lemon juice (15ml)
- 1/2 tsp lemon zest (1g)
- 1 tbsp monk fruit sweetener (12g)
- 1/4 cup shredded coconut (30g)
- 1 egg white (30g)

Instructions:

1. Preheat oven to 350°F (180°C).
2. Mix coconut and egg white, press into muffin cups to form crusts. Bake 10 minutes.
3. Mix ricotta, lemon juice, zest, and sweetener. Spoon over crusts.
4. Bake for 5 more minutes. Cool and serve.

Nutritional Facts (Per Serving): Calories: 250 | Carbs: 8g | Protein: 9g | Fat: 10g | Sugar: 2g | Fiber: 3g | Sodium: 210mg

Glycemic Index: Coconut: Low (GI = 45) | Ricotta: Low (GI = 27)

Strawberry Coconut Yogurt Bark

Prep: 10 minutes | Cook: None (Freeze: 2 hours) | Serves: 2

Ingredients:

- 1/2 cup plain Greek yogurt (120g)
- 1 tbsp monk fruit sweetener (12g)
- 2 tbsp shredded coconut (15g)
- 1/4 cup strawberries, sliced (40g)

Instructions:

1. Mix yogurt with sweetener and shredded coconut.
2. Spread the mixture on a parchment-lined tray.
3. Top with sliced strawberries.
4. Freeze for 2 hours, then break into pieces and serve.

Nutritional Facts (Per Serving): Calories: 250 | Carbs: 10g | Protein: 9g | Fat: 10g | Sugars: 3g | Fiber: 3g | Sodium: 200mg

Glycemic Index: Greek yogurt: Low (GI = 11) | Strawberries: Low (GI = 25) | Coconut: Low (GI = 45)

Banana Almond Mug Muffin

Prep: 5 minutes | Cook: 2 minutes (microwave) | Serves: 2

Ingredients:

- 1 small ripe banana, mashed (100g)
- 1/4 cup almond flour (25g)
- 1 tbsp allulose (12g)
- 1 large egg (50g)
- 1/2 tsp baking powder (2g)
- 1/4 tsp cinnamon (1g)

Instructions:

1. Mix all ingredients in a bowl until smooth.
2. Pour into a mug and microwave for 90–120 seconds.
3. Let cool slightly and serve.

Nutritional Facts (Per Serving): Calories: 250 | Carbs: 18g | Protein: 8g | Fat: 10g | Sugars: 5g | Fiber: 3g | Sodium: 200mg

Glycemic Index: Banana: Medium (GI = 51) | Almond flour: Low (GI = 10)

No-Bake Coconut Almond Bars

Prep: 10 minutes | Cook: None (Chill: 30 min) | Serves: 2

Ingredients:

- 1/2 cup shredded coconut (40g)
- 2 tbsp almond flour (20g)
- 1 tbsp almond butter (15g)
- 1 tbsp allulose (12g)
- 1 tbsp coconut oil (15ml)
- 1/2 tsp vanilla extract (2.5ml)

Instructions:

1. Mix all ingredients in a bowl until sticky and uniform.
2. Press into a small container or form bars by hand.
3. Chill in the fridge for 30 minutes until firm. Serve cold.

Nutritional Facts (Per Serving): Calories: 250 | Carbs: 9g | Protein: 8g | Fat: 10g | Sugars: 2g | Fiber: 4g | Sodium: 200mg

Glycemic Index: Coconut: Low (GI = 45) | Almond flour: Low (GI = 10) | Almond butter: Low (GI = 15)

Cinnamon Vanilla Chia Custard

Prep: 10 minutes | Cook: None (Chill: 1 hour) | Serves: 2

Ingredients:

- 1/2 cup unsweetened almond milk (120ml)
- 2 tbsp chia seeds (30g)
- 1 tbsp allulose (12g)
- 1/2 tsp vanilla extract (2.5ml)
- 1/4 tsp ground cinnamon (1g)

Instructions:

1. In a bowl, whisk almond milk, allulose, vanilla, and cinnamon.
2. Stir in chia seeds and mix well.
3. Chill for at least 1 hour until thickened. Stir before serving.

Nutritional Facts (Per Serving): Calories: 250 | Carbohydrates: 10g | Protein: 8g | Fat: 10g | Sugars: 2g | Fiber: 6g | Sodium: 100mg

Glycemic Index: Chia seeds: Low (GI = 1) | Almond milk: Low (GI = 30)

Hazelnut Cocoa Energy Truffles

Prep: 10 minutes | Cook: None (Chill: 20 minutes) | Serves: 2

Ingredients:

- 1/4 cup hazelnuts, chopped (30g)
- 1 tbsp almond flour (10g)
- 1 tbsp unsweetened cocoa powder (8g)
- 1 tbsp monk fruit sweetener (12g)
- 1 tbsp coconut oil, melted (15ml)
- 1/4 tsp vanilla extract (1.25ml)

Instructions:

1. Mix all ingredients in a bowl.
2. Form into small truffles.
3. Chill for 20 minutes before serving.

Nutritional Facts (Per Serving): Calories: 250 | Carbohydrates: 8g | Protein: 9g | Fat: 10g | Sugars: 2g | Fiber: 4g | Sodium: 180mg

Glycemic Index: Hazelnuts: Low (GI = 15) | Cocoa powder: Low (GI = 20)

Delicious Cookies, Cakes, and Treats That Fit into Your Diabetic Plan

Coconut Flour Chocolate Chip Cookies

Prep: 10 minutes | Cook: 12 minutes | Serves: 4

Ingredients:

- 1/4 cup coconut flour (30g)
- 2 tbsp dark chocolate chips (30g)
- 1 large egg (50g)
- 2 tbsp melted butter (30g)
- 1 tbsp low carb sweetener (12g)
- 1/2 tsp vanilla extract (2.5ml)
- 1/4 tsp baking soda (1g)

Instructions:

1. Preheat oven to 350°F (180°C).
2. Mix dry ingredients in bowl.
3. Add egg, butter, vanilla. Stir.
4. Drop spoonfuls on baking sheet. Bake 10–12 min.

Nutritional Facts (Per Serving): Calories: 250 | Carbohydrates: 10g | Protein: 9g | Fat: 10g | Sugars: 3g | Fiber: 5g | Sodium: 200mg

Glycemic Index: Coconut flour: Low (GI = 45) | Dark chocolate: Low (GI = 25)

Almond Flour Lemon Poppy Seed Muffins

Prep: 10 minutes | Cook: 20 minutes | Serves: 4

Ingredients:

- 1 cup almond flour (100g)
- 2 large eggs (100g)
- 2 tbsp low carb sweetener (24g)
- 1 tbsp poppy seeds (10g)
- 2 tbsp lemon juice (30ml)
- 1 tsp lemon zest (2g)
- 1/2 tsp baking powder (2g)

Instructions:

1. Preheat oven to 350°F (180°C).
2. In a bowl, mix almond flour, sweetener, poppy seeds, lemon juice, lemon zest, eggs, and baking powder.
3. Pour the batter into muffin tins and bake for 18-20 minutes.
4. Let cool before serving.

Nutritional Facts (Per Serving): Calories: 250 | Carbohydrates: 8g | Protein: 9g | Fat: 10g | Sugars: 2g | Fiber: 4g | Sodium: 200mg

Glycemic Index: Almond flour: Low (GI = 10) | Poppy seeds: Low (GI = 15) | Lemon juice: Negligible GI

Keto Blueberry Mug Cake with Almond Flour

Prep: 5 minutes | Cook: 2 minutes | Serves: 1

Ingredients:

- 1/4 cup almond flour (30g)
- 1 large egg (50g)
- 1 tbsp low carb sweetener (12g)
- 1/4 tsp baking powder (1g)
- 1/4 tsp vanilla extract (1ml)
- 2 tbsp fresh blueberries (30g)

Instructions:

1. In a microwave-safe mug, mix almond flour, sweetener, baking powder, egg, and vanilla extract until smooth.
2. Gently fold in the blueberries.
3. Microwave for 90 seconds to 2 minutes until the cake is set. Let cool slightly before serving.

Nutritional Facts (Per Serving): Calories: 250 | Carbohydrates: 9g | Protein: 9g | Fat: 10g | Sugars: 3g | Fiber: 4g | Sodium: 220mg

Glycemic Index: Almond flour: Low (GI = 10) | Blueberries: Low (GI = 25)

Low-Sugar Apple Spice Cake with Almond Flour

Prep: 10 minutes | Cook: 25 minutes | Serves: 4

Ingredients:

- 1 cup almond flour (100g)
- 1 large apple, grated (100g)
- 2 large eggs (100g)
- 2 tbsp low carb sweetener (24g)
- 1 tsp ground cinnamon (2g)
- 1/2 tsp baking powder (2g)

Instructions:

1. Preheat oven to 350°F (180°C).
2. In a bowl, mix almond flour, grated apple, sweetener, cinnamon, eggs, and baking powder.
3. Pour the batter into a greased baking dish and bake for 20-25 minutes until golden and set. Let cool before slicing.

Nutritional Facts (Per Serving): Calories: 250 | Carbohydrates: 14g | Protein: 9g | Fat: 10g | Sugars: 6g | Fiber: 5g | Sodium: 200mg

Glycemic Index: Almond flour: Low (GI = 10) | Apple: Medium (GI = 39)

Sugar-Free Pumpkin Spice Cupcakes with Cream Cheese Frosting

Prep: 15 minutes | Cook: 20 minutes | Serves: 4

Ingredients:

- 1/2 cup almond flour (50g)
- 1/2 cup pumpkin puree (120g)
- 2 tbsp low carb sweetener (24g)
- 1 large egg (50g)
- 1 tsp pumpkin pie spice (2g)
- 1/2 tsp baking powder (2g)

Ingredients for Frosting:
- 2 oz cream cheese, softened (60g)
- 1 tbsp low carb sweetener (12g)
- 1/2 tsp vanilla extract (2.5ml)

Instructions:

1. Preheat oven to 350°F (180°C).
2. In a bowl, mix almond flour, pumpkin puree, sweetener, egg, pumpkin pie spice, and baking powder until smooth.
3. Pour the batter into muffin tins and bake for 18-20 minutes. Let cool.
4. For the frosting, mix cream cheese, sweetener, and vanilla extract until smooth.
5. Frost the cupcakes and serve.

Nutritional Facts (Per Serving): Calories: 250 | Carbohydrates: 10g | Protein: 9g | Fat: 10g | Sugars: 3g | Fiber: 4g | Sodium: 230mg

Glycemic Index: Almond flour: Low (GI = 10) | Pumpkin puree: Low (GI = 50) | Cream cheese: Low (GI = 30)

Low-Carb Chocolate Coconut Cookies

Prep: 10 minutes | Cook: 12 minutes | Serves: 4

Ingredients:

- 1/2 cup almond flour (50g)
- 2 tbsp unsweetened cocoa powder (15g)
- 2 tbsp shredded coconut (14g)
- 1 large egg (50g)
- 2 tbsp low carb sweetener (24g)
- 1 tbsp coconut oil, melted (15ml)
- 1/2 tsp vanilla extract (2.5ml)

Instructions:

1. Preheat oven to 350°F (180°C).
2. In a bowl, mix almond flour, cocoa powder, shredded coconut, and sweetener.
3. Add the egg, melted coconut oil, and vanilla extract. Stir until well combined.
4. Drop spoonfuls of dough onto a baking sheet and flatten slightly.
5. Bake for 10-12 minutes. Let cool before serving.

Nutritional Facts (Per Serving): Calories: 250 | Carbohydrates: 10g | Protein: 9g | Fat: 10g | Sugars: 2g | Fiber: 5g | Sodium: 150mg

Glycemic Index: Almond flour: Low (GI = 10) | Cocoa powder: Low (GI = 20) | Coconut: Low (GI = 45)

Coconut Flour Banana Bread with Chia Seeds

Prep: 10 minutes | Cook: 25 minutes | Serves: 4

Ingredients:

- 1/4 cup coconut flour (30g)
- 1 ripe banana, mashed (100g)
- 2 large eggs (100g)
- 2 tbsp chia seeds (24g)
- 1 tbsp low carb sweetener (12g)
- 1/2 tsp baking powder (2g)
- 1/2 tsp vanilla extract (2.5ml)

Instructions:

1. Preheat oven to 350°F (180°C).
2. In a bowl, mix mashed banana, eggs, sweetener, and vanilla extract.
3. Stir in coconut flour, chia seeds, and baking powder.
4. Pour the batter into a greased loaf pan and bake for 20-25 minutes. Let cool before slicing.

Nutritional Facts (Per Serving): Calories: 250 | Carbohydrates: 20g | Protein: 9g | Fat: 10g | Sugars: 5g | Fiber: 6g | Sodium: 200mg

Glycemic Index: Coconut flour: Low (GI = 45) | Banana: Medium (GI = 51) | Chia seeds: Low (GI = 1)

Almond Flour Peanut Butter Cookies

Prep: 10 minutes | Cook: 12 minutes | Serves: 4

Ingredients:

- 1/2 cup almond flour (50g)
- 2 tbsp peanut butter (32g)
- 2 tbsp low carb sweetener (24g)
- 1 large egg (50g)
- 1/2 tsp vanilla extract (2.5ml)
- 1/4 tsp baking soda (1g)

Instructions:

1. Preheat oven to 350°F (180°C).
2. In a bowl, mix almond flour, peanut butter, sweetener, egg, vanilla extract, and baking soda until smooth.
3. Drop spoonfuls of dough onto a baking sheet and flatten slightly.
4. Bake for 10-12 minutes. Let cool before serving.

Nutritional Facts (Per Serving): Calories: 250 | Carbohydrates: 9g | Protein: 9g | Fat: 10g | Sugars: 3g | Fiber: 4g | Sodium: 200mg

Glycemic Index: Almond flour: Low (GI = 10) | Peanut butter: Low (GI = 14)

Keto-Friendly Lemon Coconut Cake

Prep: 10 minutes | Cook: 20 minutes | Serves: 4

Ingredients:

- 1/2 cup almond flour (50g)
- 1/4 cup shredded coconut (30g)
- 2 tbsp low carb sweetener (24g)
- 2 large eggs (100g)
- 2 tbsp coconut oil, melted (30ml)
- 2 tbsp lemon juice (30ml)
- 1 tsp lemon zest (2g)
- 1/2 tsp baking powder (2g)

Instructions:

1. Preheat oven to 350°F (180°C).
2. In a bowl, mix almond flour, shredded coconut, sweetener, baking powder, eggs, coconut oil, lemon juice, and lemon zest.
3. Pour the batter into a greased cake pan and bake for 18-20 minutes. Let cool before slicing.

Nutritional Facts (Per Serving): Calories: 250 | Carbohydrates: 10g | Protein: 9g | Fat: 10g | Sugars: 3g | Fiber: 5g | Sodium: 200mg

Glycemic Index: Almond flour: Low (GI = 10) | Coconut: Low (GI = 45) | Lemon juice: Negligible GI

Cinnamon and Almond Keto Cupcakes

Prep: 10 minutes | Cook: 15 minutes | Serves: 4

Ingredients:

- 1 cup almond flour (100g)
- 2 tbsp low carb sweetener (24g)
- 1/2 tsp ground cinnamon (1g)
- 2 large eggs (100g)
- 2 tbsp melted butter (30ml)
- 1/2 tsp vanilla extract (2.5ml)
- 1/2 tsp baking powder (2g)

Instructions:

1. Preheat oven to 350°F (180°C).
2. In a bowl, mix almond flour, sweetener, cinnamon, baking powder, eggs, butter, and vanilla extract.
3. Pour the batter into muffin tins and bake for 12-15 minutes.
4. Let cool before serving.

Nutritional Facts (Per Serving): Calories: 250 | Carbohydrates: 8g | Protein: 9g | Fat: 10g | Sugars: 2g | Fiber: 4g | Sodium: 220mg

Glycemic Index: Almond flour: Low (GI = 10) | Cinnamon: Negligible GI

Low-Sugar Chocolate Almond Bars

Prep: 10 minutes | Cook: 10 minutes | Serves: 4

Ingredients:

- 1/2 cup almond flour (50g)
- 2 tbsp unsweetened cocoa powder (15g)
- 2 tbsp low carb sweetener (24g)
- 2 tbsp melted butter (30ml)
- 2 oz dark chocolate, melted (60g)
- 1/2 tsp vanilla extract (2.5ml)

Instructions:

1. In a bowl, mix almond flour, cocoa powder, sweetener, melted butter, and vanilla extract.
2. Press the mixture into a baking dish and refrigerate for 30 minutes.
3. Pour melted dark chocolate over the top and refrigerate until firm. Slice into bars and serve.

Nutritional Facts (Per Serving): Calories: 250 | Carbohydrates: 9g | Protein: 8g | Fat: 10g | Sugars: 3g | Fiber: 4g | Sodium: 150mg

Glycemic Index: Almond flour: Low (GI = 10) | Dark chocolate: Low (GI = 25) | Cocoa powder: Low (GI = 20)

Almond Flour Cinnamon Rolls with Cream Cheese Icing

Prep: 15 minutes | Cook: 20 minutes | Serves: 4

Ingredients:

- 1 cup almond flour (100g)
- 2 tbsp low carb sweetener (24g)
- 1 large egg (50g)
- 1 tbsp melted butter (15ml)
- 1 tsp ground cinnamon (2g)
- 1/2 tsp baking powder (2g)

Ingredients for Icing:

- 2 oz cream cheese, softened (60g)
- 1 tbsp low carb sweetener (12g)
- 1/2 tsp vanilla extract (2.5ml)

Instructions:

1. Preheat oven to 350°F (180°C).
2. In a bowl, mix almond flour, sweetener, cinnamon, baking powder, egg, and melted butter.
3. Roll out the dough, sprinkle with more cinnamon and sweetener, then roll it up and slice into rolls.
4. Bake for 18-20 minutes until golden.
5. For the icing, mix cream cheese, sweetener, and vanilla until smooth. Spread on the cooled rolls.

Nutritional Facts (Per Serving): Calories: 250 | Carbohydrates: 8g | Protein: 9g | Fat: 10g | Sugars: 2g | Fiber: 4g | Sodium: 220mg

Glycemic Index: Almond flour: Low (GI = 10) | Cream cheese: Low (GI = 30) | Cinnamon: Negligible GI

Keto Maple Pecan Scones

Prep: 10 minutes | Cook: 15 minutes | Serves: 4

Ingredients:

- 1 cup almond flour (100g)
- 2 tbsp chopped pecans (20g)
- 2 tbsp low carb sweetener (24g)
- 1 large egg (50g)
- 1 tbsp melted butter (15ml)
- 1/2 tsp maple extract (2.5ml)
- 1/2 tsp baking powder (2g)

Instructions:

1. Preheat oven to 350°F (180°C).
2. Mix all ingredients in a bowl.
3. Shape the dough into scones and place on a baking sheet.
4. Bake for 12-15 minutes until golden.

Nutritional Facts (Per Serving): Calories: 250 | Carbohydrates: 10g | Protein: 9g | Fat: 10g | Sugars: 2g | Fiber: 5g | Sodium: 200mg

Glycemic Index: Almond flour: Low (GI = 10) | Pecans: Low (GI = 10)

Low-Sugar Apple Cinnamon Strudel with Almond Flour Crust

Prep: 15 minutes | Cook: 25 minutes | Serves: 4

Ingredients:

Ingredients for Crust:
- 1 cup almond flour (100g)
- 1 tbsp low carb sweetener (12g)
- 1 large egg (50g)
- 2 tbsp melted butter (30ml)

Ingredients for Filling:
- 1 medium apple, peeled and sliced (100g)
- 1 tsp ground cinnamon (2g)
- 1 tbsp low carb sweetener (12g)

Instructions:

1. Preheat oven to 350°F (180°C).
2. In a bowl, mix almond flour, sweetener, egg, and melted butter to form the crust dough.
3. Roll out the dough, place the apple slices in the center, and sprinkle with cinnamon and sweetener.
4. Fold the dough over the filling and bake for 20-25 minutes.

Nutritional Facts (Per Serving): Calories: 250 | Carbohydrates: 12g | Protein: 9g | Fat: 10g | Sugars: 5g | Fiber: 4g | Sodium: 200mg

Glycemic Index: Almond flour: Low (GI = 10) | Apple: Medium (GI = 39)

Avocado and Almond Flour Matcha Cake with Creamy Lime Glaze

Prep: 15 minutes | Cook: 20 minutes | Serves: 4

Ingredients:

Ingredients for Cake:
- 1/2 cup almond flour (50g)
- 1 ripe avocado, mashed (150g)
- 2 large eggs (100g)
- 2 tbsp low carb sweetener (24g)
- 1 tbsp matcha powder (5g)
- 1/2 tsp baking powder (2g)
- 1/2 tsp vanilla extract (2.5ml)

Ingredients for Creamy Lime Glaze:
- 2 oz cream cheese, softened (60g)
- 1 tbsp lime juice (15ml)
- 1 tbsp low carb sweetener (12g)
- 1/2 tsp lime zest (1g)

Instructions:

1. Preheat oven to 350°F (180°C).
2. In a bowl, mix almond flour, matcha powder, baking powder, and sweetener.
3. In another bowl, mix mashed avocado, eggs, and vanilla extract until smooth. Combine the wet and dry ingredients.
4. Pour the batter into a greased cake pan and bake for 18-20 minutes until set.
5. For the glaze, mix cream cheese, lime juice, lime zest, and sweetener until smooth.
6. Once the cake is cooled, drizzle the lime glaze on top and serve.

Nutritional Facts (Per Serving): Calories: 250 | Carbohydrates: 12g | Protein: 9g | Fat: 10g | Sugars: 3g | Fiber: 5g | Sodium: 220mg

Glycemic Index: Almond flour: Low (GI = 10) | Avocado: Negligible GI | Matcha: Low (GI = 1) | Lime juice: Negligible GI

Almond Coconut Ice Cream Bites

Prep: 10 minutes | Cook: None | Serves: 4

Ingredients:

- 1/2 cup almond butter (120g)
- 1/4 cup shredded coconut, unsweetened (30g)
- 1/2 cup coconut cream (120ml)
- 1 tbsp low carb sweetener (12g)
- 1/2 tsp vanilla extract (2.5ml)
- Pinch of salt

Instructions:

1. In a bowl, mix almond butter, coconut cream, shredded coconut, sweetener, vanilla, and salt until smooth.
2. Scoop into silicone mini muffin molds or ice cube trays.
3. Freeze for 2 hours until solid. Serve cold as a frozen treat.

Nutritional Facts (Per Serving): Calories: 250 | Carbohydrates: 10g | Protein: 9g | Fat: 10g | Sugars: 3g | Fiber: 4g | Sodium: 200mg

Glycemic Index: Almond butter: Low (GI = 15) | Coconut: Low (GI = 45) | Coconut cream: Low (GI = 40)

Orange Almond Biscotti

Prep: 15 minutes | Cook: 25 minutes | Serves: 4

Ingredients:

- 1 cup almond flour (100g)
- 1 large egg (50g)
- 2 tbsp low carb sweetener (24g)
- 1 tbsp orange zest (6g)
- 1/2 tsp vanilla extract (2.5ml)
- 1/4 tsp baking soda (1g)
- Pinch of salt

Instructions:

1. Preheat oven to 350°F (180°C).
2. Mix all ingredients into a dough. Shape into a log and place on a lined baking sheet.
3. Bake for 15 minutes, then cool for 5 minutes. Slice into biscotti strips and return to the oven for 10 more minutes until crisp.
4. Let cool completely before serving.

Nutritional Facts (Per Serving): Calories: 250 | Carbohydrates: 9g | Protein: 9g | Fat: 10g | Sugars: 2g | Fiber: 4g | Sodium: 200mg

Glycemic Index: Almond flour: Low (GI = 10) | Orange zest: Negligible GI

Vanilla Coconut Mini Donuts

Prep: 10 minutes | Cook: 15 minutes | Serves: 4

Ingredients:

- 1/2 cup almond flour (50g)
- 1/4 cup shredded coconut, unsweetened (30g)
- 2 large eggs (100g)
- 2 tbsp low carb sweetener (24g)
- 1 tbsp coconut oil, melted (15ml)
- 1 tsp vanilla extract (5ml)
- 1/2 tsp baking powder (2g)

Instructions:

1. Preheat oven to 350°F (180°C) and lightly grease a mini donut pan.
2. Mix all ingredients until smooth and pour batter into the pan.
3. Bake for 12–15 minutes until golden. Let cool before removing from the pan.

Nutritional Facts (Per Serving): Calories: 250 | Carbohydrates: 10g | Protein: 9g | Fat: 10g | Sugars: 3g | Fiber: 4g | Sodium: 200mg

Glycemic Index: Almond flour: Low (GI = 10) | Coconut: Low (GI = 45) | Vanilla extract: Negligible GI

Low-Carb Strawberry Shortcake Cups

Prep: 15 minutes | Cook: 15 minutes | Serves: 4

Ingredients:

- 1/2 cup almond flour (50g)
- 2 large eggs (100g)
- 2 tbsp low carb sweetener (24g)
- 2 tbsp whipped coconut cream (30g)
- 1/4 tsp baking powder (1g)
- 1/2 tsp vanilla extract (2.5ml)
- 1/4 cup diced strawberries (50g)

Instructions:

1. Preheat oven to 350°F (180°C).
2. Mix almond flour, eggs, sweetener, baking powder, and vanilla extract.
3. Pour into greased muffin cups and bake for 12–15 minutes until set.
4. Cool, top with strawberries and a dollop of coconut cream before serving.

Nutritional Facts (Per Serving): Calories: 250 | Carbohydrates: 10g | Protein: 9g | Fat: 10g | Sugars: 4g | Fiber: 3g | Sodium: 200mg

Glycemic Index: Almond flour: Low (GI = 10) | Strawberries: Low (GI = 25)

Mini Chocolate Hazelnut Cakes

Prep: 10 minutes | Cook: 15 minutes | Serves: 4

Ingredients:

- 1/2 cup hazelnut flour (50g)
- 2 tbsp unsweetened cocoa powder (15g)
- 2 large eggs (100g)
- 2 tbsp low carb sweetener (24g)
- 1 tbsp melted coconut oil (15ml)
- 1/2 tsp vanilla extract (2.5ml)
- 1/4 tsp baking soda (1g)

Instructions:

1. Preheat oven to 350°F (180°C).
2. Mix all ingredients until smooth and pour into greased muffin tins.
3. Bake for 12–15 minutes. Let cool before serving.

Nutritional Facts (Per Serving): Calories: 250 | Carbohydrates: 9g | Protein: 9g | Fat: 10g | Sugars: 2g | Fiber: 4g | Sodium: 200mg

Glycemic Index: Hazelnut flour: Low (GI = 15) | Cocoa powder: Low (GI = 20)

Coconut Raspberry Thumbprint Cookies

Prep: 10 minutes | Cook: 12 minutes | Serves: 4

Ingredients:

- 1/2 cup almond flour (50g)
- 2 tbsp shredded coconut (14g)
- 1 tbsp coconut oil, melted (15ml)
- 1 large egg (50g)
- 2 tbsp low carb sweetener (24g)
- 1 tbsp sugar-free raspberry jam (15g)
- 1/2 tsp vanilla extract (2.5ml)

Instructions:

1. Preheat oven to 350°F (180°C).
2. Mix almond flour, coconut, egg, sweetener, coconut oil, and vanilla until dough forms.
3. Shape into balls, press a small indentation in the center, and fill with jam.
4. Bake for 10–12 minutes until golden.

Nutritional Facts (Per Serving): Calories: 250 | Carbohydrates: 8g | Protein: 9g | Fat: 10g | Sugars: 3g | Fiber: 4g | Sodium: 180mg

Glycemic Index: Almond flour: Low (GI = 10) | Coconut: Low (GI = 45) | Raspberry jam (sugar-free): Low (GI ≈ 30)

Chocolate Zucchini Muffins with Almond Flour

Prep: 10 minutes | Cook: 20 minutes | Serves: 4

Ingredients:

- 1/2 cup almond flour (50g)
- 1/2 cup grated zucchini, squeezed dry (60g)
- 2 tbsp unsweetened cocoa powder (15g)
- 2 tbsp low carb sweetener (24g)
- 2 large eggs (100g)
- 1 tbsp melted butter (15g)
- 1/2 tsp baking powder (2g)
- 1/2 tsp vanilla extract (2.5ml)

Instructions:

1. Preheat oven to 350°F (180°C).
2. Mix all ingredients in a bowl until smooth.
3. Pour batter into muffin tins and bake for 18–20 minutes.
4. Let cool before serving.

Nutritional Facts (Per Serving): Calories: 250 | Carbohydrates: 10g | Protein: 9g | Fat: 10g | Sugars: 3g | Fiber: 4g | Sodium: 220mg

Glycemic Index: Almond flour: Low (GI = 10) | Zucchini: Low (GI = 15)

Mini Almond Butter Blondies

Prep: 10 minutes | Cook: 15 minutes | Serves: 4

Ingredients:

- 1/2 cup almond flour (50g)
- 1/4 cup almond butter (60g)
- 2 tbsp low carb sweetener (24g)
- 1 large egg (50g)
- 1/2 tsp baking powder (2g)
- 1/2 tsp vanilla extract (2.5ml)

Instructions:

1. Preheat oven to 350°F (180°C).
2. Combine all ingredients in a bowl and mix well.
3. Spoon into greased muffin cups and bake for 12–15 minutes.
4. Cool before serving.

Nutritional Facts (Per Serving): Calories: 250 | Carbohydrates: 8g | Protein: 9g | Fat: 10g | Sugars: 2g | Fiber: 4g | Sodium: 200mg

Glycemic Index: Almond flour: Low (GI = 10) | Almond butter: Low (GI = 15)

Coconut Flour Vanilla Cupcakes with Greek Yogurt Frosting

Prep: 10 minutes | Cook: 18 minutes | Serves: 4

Ingredients:

- 1/4 cup coconut flour (30g)
- 2 large eggs (100g)
- 2 tbsp low carb sweetener (24g)
- 2 tbsp coconut oil, melted (30ml)
- 1/2 tsp baking powder (2g)
- 1/2 tsp vanilla extract (2.5ml)

Instructions:

1. Preheat oven to 350°F (180°C).
2. Mix cupcake ingredients in a bowl until smooth.
3. Pour into lined muffin tins and bake for 15–18 minutes.
4. For frosting, mix yogurt, sweetener, and vanilla.
5. Cool cupcakes and frost before serving.

Nutritional Facts (Per Serving): Calories: 250 | Carbohydrates: 10g | Protein: 9g | Fat: 10g | Sugars: 3g | Fiber: 5g | Sodium: 220mg

Glycemic Index: Coconut flour: Low (GI = 45) | Greek yogurt: Low (GI = 11)

CHAPTER 6: DINNERS: Creative Salads with Diabetic-Friendly Dressings

Kale and Spinach Salad with Balsamic Vinaigrette and Feta

Prep: 10 minutes | Cook: 0 minutes | Serves: 2

Ingredients:

- 4 cups kale and spinach mix (150g)
- 1/4 cup crumbled feta cheese (30g)
- 1/4 cup sliced almonds, toasted (30g)
- 2 tbsp balsamic vinegar (30ml)
- 1 tbsp olive oil (15ml)
- 1 tsp Dijon mustard (5g)
- Salt and pepper to taste

Instructions:

1. In a large bowl, toss the kale and spinach with crumbled feta and toasted almonds.
2. In a small bowl, whisk together balsamic vinegar, olive oil, Dijon mustard, salt, and pepper.
3. Drizzle the dressing over the salad and toss to combine. Serve immediately.

Nutritional Facts (Per Serving): Calories: 350 | Sugars: 5g | Fat: 16g | Carbohydrates: 10g | Protein: 20g | Fiber: 5g | Sodium: 450mg

Glycemic Index: Kale and Spinach: Low (GI = 15) | Feta: Low (GI = 15) | Almonds: Low (GI = 10) | Balsamic vinegar: Low (GI = 15)

Zucchini Noodle Salad with Pesto and Toasted Almonds

Prep: 10 minutes | Cook: 0 minutes | Serves: 2

Ingredients:

- 2 medium zucchinis, spiralized (300g)
- 1/4 cup pesto (60g)
- 1/4 cup toasted almonds, chopped (30g)
- 1 tbsp olive oil (15ml)
- 2 tbsp grated Parmesan cheese (15g)
- Salt and pepper to taste

Instructions:

1. In a large bowl, combine spiralized zucchini with pesto and toss until well coated.
2. Top the salad with toasted almonds and grated Parmesan cheese.
3. Drizzle olive oil, season with salt and pepper, and serve fresh.

Nutritional Facts (Per Serving): Calories: 350 | Sugars: 4g | Fat: 16g | Carbohydrates: 12g | Protein: 19g | Fiber: 5g | Sodium: 480mg

Glycemic Index: Zucchini: Low (GI = 15) | Pesto: Low (GI = 15) | Almonds: Low (GI = 10)

Arugula and Grilled Shrimp Salad with Citrus Dressing

Prep: 10 minutes | Cook: 5 minutes | Serves: 2

Ingredients:

- 10 large shrimp, peeled and deveined (200g)
- 4 cups arugula (120g)
- 1/4 cup sliced cucumber (50g)
- 1/4 avocado, sliced (50g)
- 2 tbsp olive oil (30ml)
- Juice of 1 lemon (30ml)
- 1 tsp low carb sweetener (5g)
- Salt and pepper to taste

Instructions:

1. Grill shrimp over medium heat for about 2-3 minutes per side until cooked through.
2. In a small bowl, whisk together lemon juice, olive oil, sweetener, salt, and pepper to make the dressing.
3. In a large bowl, toss arugula, cucumber, and avocado.
4. Top with grilled shrimp and drizzle with citrus dressing. Serve fresh.

Nutritional Facts (Per Serving): Calories: 350 | Sugars: 4g | Fat: 15g | Carbohydrates: 12g | Protein: 22g | Fiber: 6g | Sodium: 550mg

Glycemic Index: Arugula: Low (GI = 10) | Shrimp: Low (GI = 0) | Avocado: Low (GI = 15) | Cucumber: Low (GI = 15)

Cauliflower Tabbouleh with Mint and Lemon Vinaigrette

Prep: 15 minutes | Cook: 0 minutes | Serves: 2

Ingredients:

- 2 cups grated cauliflower (300g)
- 1/4 cup chopped fresh mint (15g)
- 1/4 cup chopped parsley (15g)
- 1/4 cup diced cucumber (50g)
- 1/4 cup diced tomatoes (50g)
- 2 tbsp olive oil (30ml)
- Juice of 1 lemon (30ml)
- 1 tsp low carb sweetener (5g)
- Salt and pepper to taste

Instructions:

1. In a large bowl, combine grated cauliflower, mint, parsley, cucumber, and tomatoes.
2. In a small bowl, whisk together olive oil, lemon juice, low carb sweetener, salt, and pepper.
3. Pour the vinaigrette over the cauliflower mixture and toss to combine. Serve fresh.

Nutritional Facts (Per Serving): Calories: 350 | Sugars: 6g | Fat: 14g | Carbohydrates: 20g | Protein: 18g | Fiber: 8g | Sodium: 500mg

Glycemic Index: Cauliflower: Low (GI = 15) | Lemon: Low (GI = 15) | Cucumber: Low (GI = 15) | Tomatoes: Low (GI = 15)

Greek Salad with Grilled Halloumi and Olive Oil Dressing

Prep: 10 minutes | Cook: 5 minutes | Serves: 2

Ingredients:

- 4 oz grilled Halloumi cheese (120g)
- 2 cups mixed salad greens (80g)
- 1/4 cup sliced cucumber (50g)
- 1/4 cup diced tomatoes (50g)
- 1/4 cup Kalamata olives, pitted (30g)
- 2 tbsp olive oil (30ml)
- 1 tbsp red wine vinegar (15ml)
- 1 tsp dried oregano (5g)
- Salt and pepper to taste

Instructions:

1. Grill Halloumi over medium heat for 2-3 minutes per side until golden.
2. In a large bowl, combine salad greens, cucumber, tomatoes, and olives.
3. In a small bowl, whisk together olive oil, red wine vinegar, oregano, salt, and pepper.
4. Top the salad with grilled Halloumi and drizzle with dressing. Serve fresh.

Nutritional Facts (Per Serving): Calories: 350 | Sugars: 4g | Fat: 15g | Carbohydrates: 10g | Protein: 20g | Fiber: 5g | Sodium: 550mg

Glycemic Index: Halloumi: Low (GI = 0) | Cucumber: Low (GI = 15) | Tomatoes: Low (GI = 15) | Olives: Low (GI = 15)

Cucumber and Radish Salad with Creamy Dill Yogurt Dressing

Prep: 10 minutes | Cook: 0 minutes | Serves: 2

Ingredients:

- 1 cup sliced cucumber (120g)
- 1/2 cup sliced radishes (60g)
- 1/2 cup plain Greek yogurt (120g)
- 2 tbsp chopped fresh dill (10g)
- 1 tbsp lemon juice (15ml)
- 1 tsp low carb sweetener (5g)
- Salt and pepper to taste

Instructions:

1. In a large bowl, toss cucumber and radishes together.
2. In a small bowl, whisk Greek yogurt, dill, lemon juice, low carb sweetener, salt, and pepper to make the dressing.
3. Pour the dressing over the salad and toss to coat. Serve chilled.

Nutritional Facts (Per Serving): Calories: 350 | Sugars: 5g | Fat: 13g | Carbohydrates: 15g | Protein: 22g | Fiber: 4g | Sodium: 480mg

Glycemic Index: Cucumber: Low (GI = 15) | Radishes: Low (GI = 15) | Greek Yogurt: Low (GI = 15)

Grilled Turkey and Mixed Greens Salad with Mustard Vinaigrette

Prep: 10 minutes | Cook: 10 minutes | Serves: 2

Ingredients:

- 6 oz grilled turkey breast (170g)
- 4 cups mixed salad greens (120g)
- 1/4 cup sliced cucumber (50g)
- 1/4 cup cherry tomatoes, halved (50g)
- 2 tbsp olive oil (30ml)
- 1 tbsp Dijon mustard (15g)
- 1 tbsp apple cider vinegar (15ml)
- 1 tsp low carb sweetener (5g)
- Salt and pepper to taste

Instructions:

1. Grill turkey breast over medium heat for 4-5 minutes per side until cooked through.
2. In a small bowl, whisk together olive oil, Dijon mustard, apple cider vinegar, low carb sweetener, salt, and pepper to make the vinaigrette.
3. In a large bowl, toss mixed greens, cucumber, and cherry tomatoes.
4. Slice the grilled turkey and place on top of the salad. Drizzle with mustard vinaigrette. Serve fresh.

Nutritional Facts (Per Serving): Calories: 350 | Sugars: 4g | Fat: 14g | Carbohydrates: 12g | Protein: 22g | Fiber: 5g | Sodium: 550mg

Glycemic Index: Mixed greens: Low (GI = 10) | Turkey: Low (GI = 0) | Cucumber: Low (GI = 15) | Tomatoes: Low (GI = 15)

Spinach and Strawberry Salad with Poppy Seed Dressing

Prep: 10 minutes | Cook: 0 minutes | Serves: 2

Ingredients:

- 4 cups baby spinach (120g)
- 1/2 cup sliced strawberries (75g)
- 1/4 cup crumbled feta cheese (30g)
- 2 tbsp olive oil (30ml)
- 1 tbsp apple cider vinegar (15ml)
- 1 tsp poppy seeds (5g)
- 1 tsp low carb sweetener (5g)
- Salt and pepper to taste

Instructions:

1. In a large bowl, combine baby spinach, sliced strawberries, and crumbled feta.
2. In a small bowl, whisk together olive oil, apple cider vinegar, poppy seeds, low carb sweetener, salt, and pepper to make the dressing.
3. Drizzle the dressing over the salad and toss gently. Serve fresh.

Nutritional Facts (Per Serving): Calories: 350 | Sugars: 7g | Fat: 15g | Carbohydrates: 20g | Protein: 18g | Fiber: 6g | Sodium: 450mg

Glycemic Index: Spinach: Low (GI = 15) | Strawberries: Low (GI = 40) | Feta: Low (GI = 15)

Roasted Beet and Goat Cheese Salad with Balsamic Glaze

Prep: 10 minutes | Cook: 20 minutes | Serves: 2

Ingredients:

- 2 small beets, roasted and diced (150g)
- 4 cups arugula (120g)
- 1/4 cup crumbled goat cheese (30g)
- 2 tbsp balsamic vinegar (30ml)
- 1 tbsp olive oil (15ml)
- 1 tsp low carb sweetener (5g)
- Salt and pepper to taste

Instructions:

1. Roast beets in the oven at 400°F (200°C) for 20 minutes or until tender. Let cool and dice.
2. In a small bowl, whisk together balsamic vinegar, olive oil, low carb sweetener, salt, and pepper to make the glaze.
3. In a large bowl, toss arugula and diced beets.
4. Top with crumbled goat cheese and drizzle with balsamic glaze. Serve fresh.

Nutritional Facts (Per Serving): Calories: 350 | Sugars: 8g | Fat: 14g | Carbohydrates: 20g | Protein: 18g | Fiber: 7g | Sodium: 500mg

Glycemic Index: Beets: Medium (GI = 65) | Arugula: Low (GI = 10) | Goat cheese: Low (GI = 15)

Roasted Eggplant Salad with Tahini-Lemon Dressing

Prep: 15 minutes | Cook: 20 minutes | Serves: 2

Ingredients:

- 1 medium eggplant, cubed (250g)
- 1 tbsp olive oil (15ml)
- 2 cups mixed greens (60g)
- 1/4 cup cherry tomatoes, halved (50g)
- 1 tbsp tahini (15g)
- 1 tbsp lemon juice (15ml)
- 1 tsp low carb sweetener (5g)
- Salt and pepper to taste

Instructions:

1. Preheat oven to 400°F (200°C). Toss cubed eggplant with olive oil, salt, and pepper. Roast for 20 minutes until tender.
2. In a bowl, whisk tahini, lemon juice, sweetener, salt, and pepper.
3. Arrange mixed greens on a plate. Add roasted eggplant and cherry tomatoes.
4. Drizzle with dressing and serve.

Nutritional Facts (Per Serving): Calories: 350 | Carbs: 14g | Protein: 18g | Fat: 15g | Sugars: 5g | Fiber: 6g | Sodium: 480mg

Glycemic Index: Eggplant: Low (GI = 15) | Tahini: Low (GI = 15) | Cherry Tomatoes: Low (GI = 15)

Broccoli and Chickpea Salad with Garlic Yogurt Dressing

Prep: 10 minutes | Cook: 5 minutes | Serves: 2

Ingredients:

- 1 cup steamed broccoli florets (150g)
- 1/2 cup canned chickpeas, rinsed (120g)
- 1/2 cup plain Greek yogurt (120g)
- 1 clove garlic, minced (3g)
- 1 tbsp lemon juice (15ml)
- 1 tbsp olive oil (15ml)
- Salt and pepper to taste

Instructions:

1. Steam broccoli until tender but crisp.
2. In a bowl, whisk Greek yogurt, garlic, lemon juice, olive oil, salt, and pepper.
3. Combine broccoli and chickpeas in a bowl. Add dressing and mix well.
4. Chill and serve.

Nutritional Facts (Per Serving): Calories: 350 | Carbs: 18g | Protein: 20g | Fat: 14g | Sugars: 4g | Fiber: 7g | Sodium: 500mg

Glycemic Index: Broccoli: Low (GI = 15) | Chickpeas: Low (GI = 28) | Yogurt: Low (GI = 15)

Asian-Inspired Cabbage Salad with Sesame Ginger Dressing

Prep: 10 minutes | Cook: None | Serves: 2

Ingredients:

- 2 cups shredded Napa cabbage (140g)
- 1/2 cup shredded carrots (60g)
- 2 tbsp sesame seeds (20g)
- 1 tbsp grated ginger (6g)
- 1 tbsp soy sauce, low sodium (15ml)
- 1 tbsp rice vinegar (15ml)
- 1 tbsp olive oil (15ml)
- 1 tsp low carb sweetener (5g)

Instructions:

1. In a bowl, whisk together olive oil, soy sauce, vinegar, ginger, and sweetener to make the dressing.
2. Toss cabbage and carrots with dressing.
3. Top with sesame seeds and serve fresh.

Nutritional Facts (Per Serving): Calories: 350 | Carbs: 16g | Protein: 19g | Fat: 14g | Sugars: 5g | Fiber: 6g | Sodium: 480mg

Glycemic Index: Cabbage: Low (GI = 15) | Carrots: Low (GI = 35) | Sesame seeds: Low (GI = 10)

Avocado and Cucumber Salad with Lime-Cilantro Dressing

Prep: 10 minutes | **Cook:** 0 minutes | **Serves:** 2

Ingredients:

- 1 medium cucumber, sliced (200g)
- 1 ripe avocado, diced (150g)
- 1 tbsp chopped fresh cilantro (5g)
- Juice of 1 lime (30ml)
- 1 tbsp olive oil (15ml)
- 1 tsp low carb sweetener (5g)
- Salt and pepper to taste

Instructions:

1. In a bowl, combine cucumber and diced avocado.
2. In a small bowl, whisk together lime juice, olive oil, sweetener, cilantro, salt, and pepper.
3. Pour dressing over salad and toss gently. Serve immediately.

Nutritional Facts (Per Serving): Calories: 350 | Carbs: 10g | Protein: 18g | Fat: 16g | Sugars: 4g | Fiber: 6g | Sodium: 450mg

Glycemic Index: Cucumber: Low (GI = 15) | Avocado: Low (GI = 15) | Lime juice: Negligible GI

Roasted Cauliflower and Chickpea Salad with Tahini-Garlic Dressing

Prep: 10 minutes | **Cook:** 20 minutes | **Serves:** 2

Ingredients:

- 1 cup cauliflower florets (150g)
- 1/2 cup canned chickpeas, rinsed (120g)
- 1 tbsp olive oil (15ml)
- 1 tbsp tahini (15g)
- 1 clove garlic, minced (3g)
- 1 tbsp lemon juice (15ml)
- 1 tsp low carb sweetener (5g)
- Salt and pepper to taste

Instructions:

1. Preheat oven to 400°F (200°C). Toss cauliflower and chickpeas with half the olive oil, salt, and pepper. Roast for 20 minutes.
2. Whisk tahini, remaining olive oil, lemon juice, garlic, sweetener, salt, and pepper to make dressing.
3. Mix roasted cauliflower and chickpeas with dressing. Serve warm or chilled.

Nutritional Facts (Per Serving): Calories: 350 | Carbs: 20g | Protein: 18g | Fat: 15g | Sugars: 5g | Fiber: 7g | Sodium: 500mg

Glycemic Index: Cauliflower: Low (GI = 15) | Chickpeas: Low (GI = 28) | Tahini: Low (GI = 15)

Spinach and Avocado Salad with Warm Mushroom Vinaigrette

Prep: 10 minutes | **Cook:** 5 minutes | **Serves:** 2

Ingredients:

- 2 cups baby spinach (60g)
- 1/2 avocado, sliced (75g)
- 1/2 cup mushrooms, sliced (75g)
- 1 tbsp olive oil (15ml)
- 1 tbsp balsamic vinegar (15ml)
- 1 tsp Dijon mustard (5g)
- Salt and pepper to taste

Instructions:

1. In a skillet, sauté mushrooms in olive oil over medium heat for 4–5 minutes. Remove from heat and stir in vinegar, mustard, salt, and pepper.
2. In a bowl, toss spinach and avocado.
3. Pour warm mushroom vinaigrette over salad and toss gently. Serve immediately.

Nutritional Facts (Per Serving): Calories: 350 | Carbs: 9g | Protein: 20g | Fat: 16g | Sugars: 4g | Fiber: 6g | Sodium: 450mg

Glycemic Index: Spinach: Low (GI = 15) | Avocado: Low (GI = 15) | Mushrooms: Low (GI = 15)

Grilled Eggplant Salad with Yogurt-Tahini Dressing

Prep: 10 minutes | Cook: 10 minutes | Serves: 2

Ingredients:

- 1 medium eggplant, sliced (250g)
- 1 tbsp olive oil (15ml)
- 1/4 cup plain Greek yogurt (60g)
- 1 tbsp tahini (15g)
- 1 tbsp lemon juice (15ml)
- 1/2 tsp garlic powder (1g)
- Salt and pepper to taste

Instructions:

1. Brush eggplant slices with olive oil and grill 4–5 minutes per side.
2. In a bowl, whisk yogurt, tahini, lemon juice, garlic powder, salt, and pepper.
3. Arrange grilled eggplant on a plate and drizzle with yogurt-tahini dressing. Serve warm or chilled.

Nutritional Facts (Per Serving): Calories: 350 | Carbs: 12g | Protein: 20g | Fat: 15g | Sugars: 5g | Fiber: 6g | Sodium: 480mg

Glycemic Index: Eggplant: Low (GI = 15) | Yogurt: Low (GI = 15) | Tahini: Low (GI = 15)

Broccoli and Avocado Salad with Lemon-Garlic Dressing

Prep: 10 minutes | Cook: 5 minutes | Serves: 2

Ingredients:

- 1 cup steamed broccoli florets (150g)
- 1/2 avocado, diced (75g)
- 1 tbsp olive oil (15ml)
- 1 tbsp lemon juice (15ml)
- 1 clove garlic, minced (3g)
- Salt and pepper to taste

Instructions:

1. Steam broccoli until just tender. Let cool slightly.
2. In a small bowl, whisk olive oil, lemon juice, garlic, salt, and pepper.
3. In a bowl, combine broccoli and avocado, then drizzle with dressing. Toss gently and serve.

Nutritional Facts (Per Serving): Calories: 350 | Carbs: 10g | Protein: 20g | Fat: 16g | Sugars: 3g | Fiber: 6g | Sodium: 460mg

Glycemic Index: Broccoli: Low (GI = 15) | Avocado: Low (GI = 15) | Lemon juice: Negligible GI

Red Cabbage Slaw with Apple Cider Mustard Dressing

Prep: 10 minutes | Cook: 0 minutes | Serves: 2

Ingredients:

- 2 cups shredded red cabbage (150g)
- 1/4 cup grated carrot (30g)
- 1 tbsp olive oil (15ml)
- 1 tbsp apple cider vinegar (15ml)
- 1 tsp Dijon mustard (5g)
- Salt and pepper to taste

Instructions:

1. In a large bowl, combine shredded cabbage and grated carrot.
2. In a small bowl, whisk olive oil, apple cider vinegar, Dijon mustard, salt, and pepper.
3. Pour dressing over slaw and toss to coat evenly. Let sit 5 minutes before serving.

Nutritional Facts (Per Serving): Calories: 350 | Carbs: 14g | Protein: 20g | Fat: 14g | Sugars: 5g | Fiber: 5g | Sodium: 450mg

Glycemic Index: Red cabbage: Low (GI = 15) | Carrot: Low (GI = 35) | Apple cider vinegar: Negligible GI

Simple, Satisfying Meals for Busy Evenings

Grilled Chicken Salad with Cauli Rice & Tahini

Prep: 15 minutes | **Cook:** 10 minutes | **Serves:** 2

Ingredients:

- 1 cup cauliflower rice (150g)
- 6 oz grilled chicken breast, sliced (170g)
- 4 cups arugula (120g)
- 1 tbsp tahini (15g)
- Juice of 1 lemon (30ml)
- 1 tbsp olive oil (15ml)
- 1 tsp low carb sweetener (5g)
- Salt and pepper to taste

Instructions:

1. Grill chicken 4–5 min/side, slice.
2. Whisk tahini, lemon, oil, sweetener, salt, pepper.
3. Toss arugula & cauliflower rice.
4. Top with chicken, drizzle dressing. Serve.

Nutritional Facts (Per Serving): Calories: 350 | Sugars: 3g | Fat: 14g | Carbohydrates: 15g | Protein: 22g | Fiber: 6g | Sodium: 480mg

Glycemic Index: Cauliflower: Low (GI = 15) | Chicken: Low (GI = 0) | Arugula: Low (GI = 10)

Eggplant and Mushroom Stir-Fry with Brown Rice

Prep: 10 minutes | **Cook:** 15 minutes | **Serves:** 2

Ingredients:

- 1 medium eggplant, diced (200g)
- 1 cup sliced mushrooms (100g)
- 1 cup cooked brown rice (150g)
- 2 tbsp olive oil (30ml)
- 1 tbsp soy sauce (15ml)
- 1 tsp low carb sweetener (5g)
- 1 tsp minced garlic (5g)
- Salt and pepper to taste

Instructions:

1. Heat olive oil in a pan over medium heat. Add diced eggplant and cook for 5 minutes.
2. Add mushrooms, garlic, and soy sauce. Stir-fry for another 5 minutes until vegetables are tender.
3. Stir in low carb sweetener, salt, and pepper.
4. Serve the stir-fried vegetables over cooked brown rice.

Nutritional Facts (Per Serving): Calories: 350 | Sugars: 6g | Fat: 14g | Carbohydrates: 30g | Protein: 18g | Fiber: 7g | Sodium: 550mg

Glycemic Index: Eggplant: Low (GI = 15) | Mushrooms: Low (GI = 15) | Brown rice: Medium (GI = 50)

Portobello Mushrooms Stuffed with Quinoa

Prep: 10 minutes | **Cook:** 20 minutes | **Serves:** 2

Ingredients:

- 4 large portobello mushrooms (300g)
- 1 cup cooked quinoa (150g)
- 1/4 cup crumbled feta cheese (30g)
- 2 tbsp olive oil (30ml)
- 1 tbsp chopped fresh parsley (15g)
- 1 tbsp lemon juice (15ml)
- 1 clove garlic, minced (5g)
- Salt and pepper to taste

Instructions:

1. Preheat the oven to 375°F (190°C). Brush mushrooms with olive oil and season with salt and pepper.
2. In a bowl, mix cooked quinoa, feta, parsley, lemon juice, garlic, salt, and pepper.
3. Stuff each mushroom cap with the quinoa mixture.
4. Bake for 15-20 minutes until mushrooms are tender. Serve warm.

Nutritional Facts (Per Serving): Calories: 350 | Sugars: 4g | Fat: 14g | Carbohydrates: 22g | Protein: 18g | Fiber: 6g | Sodium: 500mg

Glycemic Index: Quinoa: Medium (GI = 53) | Mushrooms: Low (GI = 15) | Feta: Low (GI = 15)

Creamy Amaranth Porridge with Toasted Almonds and Fresh Herbs

Prep: 5 minutes | Cook: 15 minutes | Serves: 2

Ingredients:

- 1/2 cup amaranth (80g)
- 1 1/2 cups water (360ml)
- 1/4 cup toasted almonds, chopped (30g)
- 2 tbsp olive oil (30ml)
- 1 tbsp chopped fresh parsley (15g)
- 1/2 tsp low carb sweetener (2g)
- Salt to taste

Instructions:

1. In a pot, bring water to a boil and add amaranth. Simmer for 15 minutes until the grains are tender and creamy.
2. Stir in olive oil, toasted almonds, parsley, low carb sweetener, and salt.
3. Serve warm, garnished with extra fresh herbs if desired.

Nutritional Facts (Per Serving): Calories: 350 | Sugars: 2g | Fat: 15g | Carbohydrates: 28g | Protein: 18g | Fiber: 5g | Sodium: 400mg

Glycemic Index: Amaranth: Medium (GI = 50) | Almonds: Low (GI = 10)

Cauliflower Steaks with Garlic and Herb Quinoa

Prep: 10 minutes | Cook: 20 minutes | Serves: 2

Ingredients:

- 1 large cauliflower, cut into 2 thick steaks (300g)
- 1 cup cooked quinoa (150g)
- 2 tbsp olive oil (30ml)
- 1 clove garlic, minced (5g)
- 1 tbsp chopped fresh rosemary (15g)
- 1 tbsp lemon juice (15ml)
- Salt and pepper to taste

Instructions:

1. Preheat the oven to 400°F (200°C). Brush cauliflower steaks with olive oil, garlic, rosemary, salt, and pepper.
2. Roast cauliflower steaks for 20 minutes, flipping halfway through, until tender and golden.
3. In a bowl, toss cooked quinoa with olive oil, lemon juice, salt, and pepper.
4. Serve roasted cauliflower steaks over the quinoa.

Nutritional Facts (Per Serving): Calories: 350 | Sugars: 3g | Fat: 14g | Carbohydrates: 24g | Protein: 18g | Fiber: 6g | Sodium: 480mg

Glycemic Index: Cauliflower: Low (GI = 15) | Quinoa: Medium (GI = 53)

Buckwheat Porridge with Roasted Vegetables and Feta

Prep: 10 minutes | Cook: 20 minutes | Serves: 2

Ingredients:

- 1/2 cup uncooked buckwheat (85g)
- 1 cup water (240ml)
- 1/2 cup diced bell pepper (75g)
- 1/2 cup diced zucchini (75g)
- 1/4 cup crumbled feta cheese (30g)
- 1 tbsp olive oil (15ml)
- 1 clove garlic, minced (5g)
- Salt and pepper to taste

Instructions:

1. Cook buckwheat in 1 cup of water until tender, about 15 minutes.
2. In a skillet, heat olive oil over medium heat. Add bell pepper, zucchini, and garlic. Sauté until vegetables are tender, about 5-7 minutes.
3. Mix cooked buckwheat with roasted vegetables and top with crumbled feta. Season with salt and pepper. Serve warm.

Nutritional Facts (Per Serving): Calories: 350 | Sugars: 4g | Fat: 14g | Carbohydrates: 26g | Protein: 18g | Fiber: 6g | Sodium: 500mg

Glycemic Index: Buckwheat: Medium (GI = 54) | Feta: Low (GI = 15) | Zucchini: Low (GI = 15)

Ratatouille

Prep: 15 minutes | Cook: 30 minutes | Serves: 2

Ingredients:

- 1/2 cup diced eggplant (75g)
- 1/2 cup diced zucchini (75g)
- 1/2 cup diced bell pepper (75g)
- 1/4 cup diced tomatoes (50g)
- 1 tbsp olive oil (15ml)
- 1 clove garlic, minced (5g)
- 1 tsp fresh thyme (5g)
- Salt and pepper to taste

Instructions:

1. Heat olive oil in a large skillet over medium heat. Add garlic and sauté for 1 minute.
2. Add eggplant, zucchini, and bell pepper. Cook for 10 minutes, stirring occasionally.
3. Add tomatoes and thyme. Continue cooking for another 15-20 minutes until vegetables are tender.
4. Season with salt and pepper and serve warm.

Nutritional Facts (Per Serving): Calories: 350 | Sugars: 6g | Fat: 14g | Carbohydrates: 26g | Protein: 18g | Fiber: 7g | Sodium: 480mg

Glycemic Index: Eggplant: Low (GI = 15) | Zucchini: Low (GI = 15) | Tomatoes: Low (GI = 15)

Pilaf with Brown Rice

Prep: 10 minutes | Cook: 25 minutes | Serves: 2

Ingredients:

- 1/2 cup uncooked brown rice (90g)
- 1 cup chicken broth (240ml)
- 1/4 cup diced carrots (40g)
- 1/4 cup diced onion (40g)
- 1/4 cup cooked chicken breast, diced (60g)
- 1 tbsp olive oil (15ml)
- 1/2 tsp ground cumin (2g)
- Salt and pepper to taste

Instructions:

1. Heat olive oil in a large pan over medium heat. Add carrots and onions, sauté for 5 minutes.
2. Add brown rice and cumin, stir to coat. Pour in chicken broth and bring to a boil.
3. Reduce heat to low, cover, and simmer for 20 minutes until rice is tender.
4. Stir in cooked chicken, season with salt and pepper, and serve warm.

Nutritional Facts (Per Serving): Calories: 350 | Sugars: 3g | Fat: 14g | Carbohydrates: 28g | Protein: 20g | Fiber: 5g | Sodium: 480mg

Glycemic Index: Brown rice: Medium (GI = 50) | Carrots: Medium (GI = 35) | Chicken: Low (GI = 0)

Zucchini Noodles with Pesto and Sautéed Mushrooms

Prep: 10 minutes | Cook: 10 minutes | Serves: 2

Ingredients:

- 2 medium zucchinis, spiralized (300g)
- 1/2 cup sliced mushrooms (75g)
- 1/4 cup pesto (60g)
- 1 tbsp olive oil (15ml)
- 1 clove garlic, minced (5g)
- Salt and pepper to taste

Instructions:

1. Heat olive oil in a skillet over medium heat. Add mushrooms and garlic, sauté for 5 minutes until tender.
2. In a large bowl, toss zucchini noodles with pesto.
3. Add sautéed mushrooms to the noodles and toss again. Season with salt and pepper to taste. Serve immediately.

Nutritional Facts (Per Serving): Calories: 350 | Sugars: 4g | Fat: 15g | Carbohydrates: 20g | Protein: 18g | Fiber: 5g | Sodium: 450mg

Glycemic Index: Zucchini: Low (GI = 15) | Mushrooms: Low (GI = 15) | Pesto: Low (GI = 15)

Stuffed Bell Peppers with Ground Turkey and Zucchini

Prep: 15 minutes | Cook: 25 minutes | Serves: 2

Ingredients:

- 2 medium bell peppers, halved and seeded (300g)
- 6 oz ground turkey (170g)
- 1/2 small zucchini, diced (75g)
- 1 small onion, diced (70g)
- 1 clove garlic, minced (5g)
- 1 tbsp olive oil (15ml)
- 1 tsp dried oregano (2g)
- Salt and pepper to taste

Instructions:

1. Preheat oven to 375°F (190°C).
2. Heat olive oil in a pan, sauté onion and garlic for 2 minutes. Add ground turkey, cook until browned.
3. Stir in zucchini, oregano, salt, and pepper. Cook for 3–4 minutes.
4. Stuff bell pepper halves with the mixture and place in a baking dish.
5. Bake for 20–25 minutes until peppers are tender. Serve hot.

Nutritional Facts (Per Serving): Calories: 350 | Carbohydrates: 16g | Protein: 22g | Fat: 14g | Sugars: 6g | Fiber: 5g | Sodium: 480mg

Glycemic Index: Bell peppers: Low (GI = 15) | Zucchini: Low (GI = 15) | Turkey: Low (GI = 0)

Lentil and Vegetable Skillet with Fresh Herbs

Prep: 10 minutes | Cook: 20 minutes | Serves: 2

Ingredients:

- 1/2 cup cooked green lentils (100g)
- 1/2 cup chopped eggplant (75g)
- 1/2 cup chopped zucchini (75g)
- 1/4 cup diced tomatoes (50g)
- 1 tbsp olive oil (15ml)
- 1 clove garlic, minced (5g)
- 1 tbsp chopped parsley (5g)
- Salt and pepper to taste

Instructions:

1. Heat olive oil in a skillet over medium heat. Sauté garlic, eggplant, and zucchini for 5 minutes.
2. Add tomatoes and lentils, season with salt and pepper. Simmer for 10 minutes, stirring occasionally.
3. Stir in fresh parsley and serve warm.

Nutritional Facts (Per Serving): Calories: 350 | Carbohydrates: 28g | Protein: 18g | Fat: 14g | Sugars: 5g | Fiber: 7g | Sodium: 450mg

Glycemic Index: Lentils: Low (GI = 32) | Eggplant: Low (GI = 15) | Zucchini: Low (GI = 15)

Tofu and Cabbage Stir-Fry with Ginger-Garlic Sauce

Prep: 10 minutes | Cook: 15 minutes | Serves: 2

Ingredients:

- 6 oz firm tofu, cubed (170g)
- 2 cups shredded green cabbage (150g)
- 1 small carrot, julienned (50g)
- 1 tbsp olive oil (15ml)
- 1 tbsp soy sauce (15ml)
- 1 tsp grated ginger (3g)
- 1 clove garlic, minced (5g)
- Salt and pepper to taste

Instructions:

1. Heat oil in a pan over medium heat. Add tofu cubes and cook until golden on all sides, about 6–7 minutes.
2. Add cabbage, carrot, garlic, ginger, and soy sauce. Stir-fry for 5–7 minutes until vegetables are tender.
3. Season with salt and pepper. Serve warm.

Nutritional Facts (Per Serving): Calories: 350 | Carbohydrates: 18g | Protein: 22g | Fat: 14g | Sugars: 4g | Fiber: 6g | Sodium: 480mg

Glycemic Index: Tofu: Low (GI = 15) | Cabbage: Low (GI = 15) | Carrot: Medium (GI = 47)

Egg and Cauliflower Skillet with Baby Spinach

Prep: 10 minutes | Cook: 15 minutes | Serves: 2

Ingredients:

- 4 large eggs (200g)
- 1 cup cauliflower rice (150g)
- 1 cup baby spinach (30g)
- 1 tbsp olive oil (15ml)
- 1 clove garlic, minced (5g)
- 1/2 tsp paprika (1g)
- Salt and pepper to taste

Instructions:

1. Heat olive oil in a nonstick skillet over medium heat. Add garlic and cauliflower rice. Sauté for 5 minutes.
2. Stir in baby spinach and cook until wilted, about 1–2 minutes.
3. Make four wells in the mixture and crack an egg into each. Cover and cook 6–8 minutes until eggs are set.
4. Season with paprika, salt, and pepper. Serve hot.

Nutritional Facts (Per Serving): Calories: 350 | Carbohydrates: 10g | Protein: 22g | Fat: 14g | Sugars: 2g | Fiber: 4g | Sodium: 450mg

Glycemic Index: Eggs: Negligible GI | Cauliflower: Low (GI = 15) | Spinach: Low (GI = 15)

Stuffed Zucchini Boats with Mushrooms and Feta

Prep: 15 minutes | Cook: 20 minutes | Serves: 2

Ingredients:

- 2 medium zucchinis, halved lengthwise (300g)
- 1 cup chopped mushrooms (100g)
- 1/4 cup crumbled feta cheese (30g)
- 1 tbsp olive oil (15ml)
- 1 clove garlic, minced (5g)
- 1 tbsp chopped parsley (5g)
- Salt and pepper to taste

Instructions:

1. Preheat oven to 375°F (190°C). Scoop out centers of zucchinis to create boats.
2. Sauté garlic and mushrooms in olive oil for 5–6 minutes until tender. Stir in parsley, salt, and pepper.
3. Fill zucchini boats with the mushroom mixture, top with feta.
4. Place in a baking dish and bake for 15–20 minutes. Serve warm.

Nutritional Facts (Per Serving): Calories: 350 | Carbohydrates: 12g | Protein: 18g | Fat: 14g | Sugars: 4g | Fiber: 5g | Sodium: 480mg

Glycemic Index: Zucchini: Low (GI = 15) | Mushrooms: Low (GI = 15) | Feta: Low (GI = 15)

Tempeh Stir-Fry with Snow Peas and Ginger

Prep: 10 minutes | Cook: 10 minutes | Serves: 2

Ingredients:

- 6 oz tempeh, sliced (170g)
- 1 cup snow peas (100g)
- 1/2 red bell pepper, sliced (75g)
- 1 tbsp olive oil (15ml)
- 1 tsp grated ginger (3g)
- 1 tbsp low-sodium soy sauce (15ml)
- Salt and pepper to taste

Instructions:

1. Heat olive oil in a large pan over medium-high heat. Add tempeh and cook until golden, about 5 minutes.
2. Add bell pepper, snow peas, ginger, and soy sauce. Stir-fry for 4–5 minutes.
3. Season with salt and pepper. Serve immediately.

Nutritional Facts (Per Serving): Calories: 350 | Carbohydrates: 14g | Protein: 22g | Fat: 14g | Sugars: 5g | Fiber: 6g | Sodium: 480mg

Glycemic Index: Tempeh: Low (GI = 15) | Snow peas: Low (GI = 15) | Bell pepper: Low (GI = 15)

Baked Tofu with Steamed Broccoli and Tahini Sauce

Prep: 10 minutes | Cook: 20 minutes | Serves: 2

Ingredients:

- 6 oz firm tofu, cubed (170g)
- 2 cups broccoli florets (150g)
- 1 tbsp olive oil (15ml)
- 1 tbsp tahini (15g)
- 1 tbsp lemon juice (15ml)
- 1 tsp low carb sweetener (5g)
- Salt and pepper to taste

Instructions:

1. Preheat oven to 375°F (190°C). Toss tofu with olive oil, salt, and pepper. Bake for 20 minutes, turning once.
2. Steam broccoli until tender, about 5–6 minutes.
3. In a small bowl, mix tahini, lemon juice, sweetener, and a splash of warm water to create a sauce.
4. Serve tofu with broccoli and drizzle with tahini sauce.

Nutritional Facts (Per Serving): Calories: 350 | Carbohydrates: 12g | Protein: 22g | Fat: 14g | Sugars: 3g | Fiber: 5g | Sodium: 480mg

Glycemic Index: Tofu: Low (GI = 15) | Broccoli: Low (GI = 15) | Tahini: Low (GI = 35)

Stuffed Bell Peppers with Ground Turkey and Quinoa

Prep: 15 minutes | Cook: 25 minutes | Serves: 2

Ingredients:

- 2 medium bell peppers, halved and seeded (200g)
- 6 oz ground turkey (170g)
- 1/2 cup cooked quinoa (75g)
- 1/4 cup diced tomatoes (50g)
- 1 tbsp olive oil (15ml)
- 1 clove garlic, minced (5g)
- 1 tsp dried basil (2g)
- Salt and pepper to taste

Instructions:

1. Preheat oven to 375°F (190°C).
2. Sauté garlic and ground turkey in olive oil for 5–6 minutes. Add cooked quinoa, tomatoes, basil, salt, and pepper.
3. Fill bell pepper halves with mixture. Place in a baking dish and bake for 20–25 minutes.
4. Serve warm.

Nutritional Facts (Per Serving): Calories: 350 | Carbohydrates: 18g | Protein: 22g | Fat: 14g | Sugars: 5g | Fiber: 6g | Sodium: 500mg

Glycemic Index: Bell pepper: Low (GI = 15) | Quinoa: Medium (GI = 53) | Tomatoes: Low (GI = 15)

Cabbage Stir-Fry with Eggs and Carrots

Prep: 10 minutes | Cook: 10 minutes | Serves: 2

Ingredients:

- 2 cups shredded cabbage (150g)
- 2 medium carrots, julienned (120g)
- 2 large eggs (100g)
- 1 tbsp olive oil (15ml)
- 1 tsp low-sodium soy sauce (5ml)
- Salt and pepper to taste

Instructions:

1. Heat olive oil in a skillet over medium heat. Sauté carrots and cabbage for 5–6 minutes until softened.
2. Push vegetables to the side. Crack in the eggs and scramble until set. Mix with vegetables.
3. Add soy sauce, salt, and pepper. Stir and serve hot.

Nutritional Facts (Per Serving): Calories: 350 | Carbohydrates: 16g | Protein: 18g | Fat: 14g | Sugars: 5g | Fiber: 5g | Sodium: 450mg

Glycemic Index: Cabbage: Low (GI = 15) | Carrots: Medium (GI = 35) | Eggs: Negligible GI

Fish and Seafood

Grilled Shrimp and Asparagus Salad with Garlic-Lemon Dressing

Prep: 10 minutes | Cook: 10 minutes | Serves: 2

Ingredients:

- 8 large shrimp, peeled and deveined (200g)
- 8 asparagus spears, trimmed (150g)
- 4 cups mixed salad greens (120g)
- 1 tbsp olive oil (15ml)
- Juice of 1 lemon (30ml)
- 1 clove garlic, minced (5g)
- Salt and pepper to taste

Instructions:

1. Grill shrimp & asparagus 4–5 min.
2. In a small bowl, whisk together olive oil, lemon juice, garlic, salt, and pepper to make the dressing.
3. In a large bowl, toss salad greens with grilled shrimp and asparagus. Drizzle with garlic-lemon dressing and serve immediately.

Nutritional Facts (Per Serving): Calories: 350 | Sugars: 3g | Fat: 14g | Carbohydrates: 12g | Protein: 22g | Fiber: 5g | Sodium: 500mg

Glycemic Index: Shrimp: Low (GI = 0) | Asparagus: Low (GI = 15) | Salad greens: Low (GI = 10)

Baked Salmon with Broccoli and Lemon Dill Sauce

Prep: 10 minutes | Cook: 15 minutes | Serves: 2

Ingredients:

- 2 salmon fillets (6 oz each) (170g each)
- 2 cups broccoli florets (200g)
- 2 tbsp olive oil (30ml)
- Juice of 1 lemon (30ml)
- 1 tbsp fresh dill, chopped (15g)
- 1 clove garlic, minced (5g)
- Salt and pepper to taste

Instructions:

1. Preheat oven to 400°F (200°C). Place salmon and broccoli on a baking sheet. Drizzle with olive oil, season with salt and pepper, and bake for 12-15 minutes.
2. In a small bowl, whisk together lemon juice, dill, and garlic to make the sauce.
3. Serve the baked salmon and broccoli with the lemon dill sauce drizzled on top.

Nutritional Facts (Per Serving): Calories: 350 | Sugars: 2g | Fat: 15g | Carbohydrates: 10g | Protein: 22g | Fiber: 4g | Sodium: 480mg

Glycemic Index: Salmon: Negligible GI (no carbs) | Broccoli: Low (GI = 15)

Tuna Niçoise Salad with Hard-Boiled Eggs and Olive Oil

Prep: 10 minutes | Cook: 8 minutes | Serves: 2

Ingredients:

- 1 can tuna in water, drained (5 oz) (140g)
- 2 hard-boiled eggs, halved (100g)
- 4 cups mixed salad greens (120g)
- 1/4 cup cherry tomatoes, halved (50g)
- 1/4 cup sliced cucumber (50g)
- 1 tbsp olive oil (15ml)
- 1 tsp Dijon mustard (5g)
- 1 tbsp lemon juice (15ml)
- Salt and pepper to taste

Instructions:

1. In a small bowl, whisk together olive oil, Dijon mustard, lemon juice, salt, and pepper to make the dressing.
2. In a large bowl, arrange salad greens, tuna, hard-boiled eggs, cherry tomatoes, and cucumber.
3. Drizzle with the dressing and serve immediately.

Nutritional Facts (Per Serving): Calories: 350 | Sugars: 3g | Fat: 15g | Carbohydrates: 10g | Protein: 22g | Fiber: 5g | Sodium: 500mg

Glycemic Index: Tuna: Low (GI = 0) | Eggs: Low (GI = 0) | Salad greens: Low (GI = 10) | Tomatoes: Low (GI = 15)

Baked Cod with Roasted Brussels Sprouts

Prep: 10 minutes | Cook: 20 minutes | Serves: 2

Ingredients:

- 2 cod fillets (6 oz each) (170g each)
- 2 cups Brussels sprouts, halved (200g)
- 2 tbsp olive oil (30ml)
- Juice of 1/2 lemon (15ml)
- 1 clove garlic, minced (5g)
- Salt and pepper to taste

Instructions:

1. Preheat oven to 400°F (200°C). Toss Brussels sprouts with 1 tbsp olive oil, salt, and pepper. Roast for 15 minutes.
2. While the Brussels sprouts are roasting, season cod fillets with lemon juice, garlic, salt, and pepper.
3. Place cod fillets on the same baking sheet with Brussels sprouts and bake for another 10-12 minutes until the fish is cooked through.
4. Serve cod with the roasted Brussels sprouts.

Nutritional Facts (Per Serving): Calories: 350 | Sugars: 3g | Fat: 15g | Carbohydrates: 12g | Protein: 22g | Fiber: 5g | Sodium: 450mg

Glycemic Index: Cod: Low (GI = 0) | Brussels Sprouts: Low (GI = 15)

Seared Tuna Steak with Avocado and Cucumber Salad

Prep: 10 minutes | Cook: 5 minutes | Serves: 2

Ingredients:

- 2 tuna steaks (5 oz each) (140g each)
- 1/2 avocado, diced (75g)
- 1/2 cucumber, sliced (75g)
- 1 tbsp olive oil (15ml)
- Juice of 1 lime (15ml)
- Salt and pepper to taste

Instructions:

1. Heat 1 tbsp olive oil in a skillet over medium-high heat. Sear tuna steaks for 2-3 minutes per side until desired doneness.
2. In a bowl, combine diced avocado, cucumber, lime juice, salt, and pepper to make the salad.
3. Serve the seared tuna with the avocado and cucumber salad.

Nutritional Facts (Per Serving): Calories: 350 | Sugars: 2g | Fat: 15g | Carbohydrates: 10g | Protein: 22g | Fiber: 5g | Sodium: 400mg

Glycemic Index: Tuna: Low (GI = 0) | Avocado: Low (GI = 15) | Cucumber: Low (GI = 15)

Herb-Crusted Halibut with Cauliflower Mash

Prep: 10 minutes | Cook: 15 minutes | Serves: 2

Ingredients:

- 2 halibut fillets (6 oz each) (170g each)
- 1/2 cup almond flour (50g)
- 1 tbsp fresh parsley, chopped (15g)
- 1 tbsp olive oil (15ml)
- 2 cups cauliflower florets (200g)
- 2 tbsp unsweetened almond milk (30ml)
- 1 clove garlic, minced (5g)
- Salt and pepper to taste

Instructions:

1. Preheat oven to 375°F (190°C). Mix almond flour, parsley, salt, and pepper in a bowl. Coat the halibut fillets with this mixture.
2. Heat 1 tbsp olive oil in a skillet over medium heat. Sear halibut for 2 minutes per side, then transfer to the oven to bake for 10 minutes.
3. Meanwhile, steam cauliflower until tender. Mash with almond milk, garlic, salt, and pepper.
4. Serve the herb-crusted halibut with the cauliflower mash.

Nutritional Facts (Per Serving): Calories: 350 | Sugars: 2g | Fat: 15g | Carbohydrates: 14g | Protein: 22g | Fiber: 6g | Sodium: 480mg

Glycemic Index: Halibut: Low (GI = 0) | Cauliflower: Low (GI = 15) | Almond flour: Low (GI = 10)

Broiled Mackerel with Sautéed Spinach

Prep: 10 minutes | Cook: 15 minutes | Serves: 2

Ingredients:

- 2 mackerel fillets (6 oz each) (170g each)
- 1 tbsp olive oil (15ml)
- 2 cups fresh spinach (60g)
- 1 clove garlic, minced (5g)
- Juice of 1/2 lemon (15ml)
- Salt and pepper to taste

Instructions:

1. Preheat the broiler. Season mackerel fillets with lemon juice, salt, and pepper.
2. Broil mackerel for 5-6 minutes until the fish is cooked through.
3. Meanwhile, heat olive oil in a skillet over medium heat. Add garlic and sauté for 1 minute.
4. Add spinach and cook for 2-3 minutes until wilted.
5. Serve the broiled mackerel with the sautéed spinach.

Nutritional Facts (Per Serving): Calories: 350 | Sugars: 2g | Fat: 15g | Carbohydrates: 8g | Protein: 22g | Fiber: 4g | Sodium: 450mg

Glycemic Index: Mackerel: Low (GI = 0) | Spinach: Low (GI = 15)

Baked Flounder with Broccoli and Cauliflower

Prep: 10 minutes | Cook: 20 minutes | Serves: 2

Ingredients:

- 2 flounder fillets (5 oz each) (140g each)
- 1 cup broccoli florets (100g)
- 1 cup cauliflower florets (100g)
- 1 tbsp olive oil (15ml)
- Juice of 1/2 lemon (15ml)
- 1 clove garlic, minced (5g)
- Salt and pepper to taste

Instructions:

1. Preheat oven to 375°F (190°C). Season flounder fillets with lemon juice, garlic, salt, and pepper.
2. Toss broccoli and cauliflower with olive oil, salt, and pepper.
3. Place flounder and vegetables on a baking sheet. Bake for 15-20 minutes until the fish is cooked through and vegetables are tender.
4. Serve the baked flounder with roasted broccoli and cauliflower.

Nutritional Facts (Per Serving): Calories: 350 | Sugars: 3g | Fat: 14g | Carbohydrates: 12g | Protein: 22g | Fiber: 5g | Sodium: 480mg

Glycemic Index: Flounder: Low (GI = 0) | Broccoli: Low (GI = 15) | Cauliflower: Low (GI = 15)

Grilled Calamari with Lemon and Arugula Salad

Prep: 10 minutes | Cook: 5 minutes | Serves: 2

Ingredients:

- 8 oz calamari, cleaned (230g)
- 4 cups arugula (120g)
- Juice of 1 lemon (30ml)
- 1 tbsp olive oil (15ml)
- 1 clove garlic, minced (5g)
- Salt and pepper to taste

Instructions:

1. Preheat the grill to medium heat. Toss calamari with olive oil, garlic, salt, and pepper.
2. Grill calamari for 2-3 minutes per side until tender.
3. In a large bowl, toss arugula with lemon juice, salt, and pepper.
4. Serve the grilled calamari on top of the arugula salad.

Nutritional Facts (Per Serving): Calories: 350 | Sugars: 2g | Fat: 14g | Carbohydrates: 10g | Protein: 22g | Fiber: 4g | Sodium: 450mg

Glycemic Index: Calamari: Low (GI = 0) | Arugula: Low (GI = 10)

Grilled Octopus with Arugula and Olive Oil

Prep: 15 minutes | Cook: 40 minutes | Serves: 2

Ingredients:

- 200g octopus, cleaned
- 4 cups arugula (120g)
- 2 tbsp olive oil (30ml)
- Juice of 1 lemon (30ml)
- 1 clove garlic, minced (5g)
- Salt and pepper to taste

Instructions:

1. Boil octopus in salted water for 30 minutes until tender. Drain and pat dry.
2. Brush with 1 tbsp olive oil and grill for 3–4 minutes per side until slightly charred.
3. Toss arugula with remaining olive oil, lemon juice, garlic, salt, and pepper.
4. Slice grilled octopus and serve over dressed arugula.

Nutritional Facts (Per Serving): Calories: 350 | Carbohydrates: 10g | Protein: 22g | Fat: 14g | Sugars: 2g | Fiber: 4g | Sodium: 500mg

Glycemic Index: Octopus: Low (GI = 0) | Arugula: Low (GI = 10)

Roasted Salmon Cakes with Yogurt Dill Sauce

Prep: 10 minutes | Cook: 20 minutes | Serves: 2

Ingredients:

- 1 can wild salmon, drained (170g)
- 1 egg (50g)
- 1/4 cup almond flour (30g)
- 1 tbsp chopped fresh dill (5g)
- 1/2 small onion, finely chopped (40g)
- Salt and pepper to taste
- 1/4 cup plain Greek yogurt (60g)
- 1 tbsp lemon juice (15ml)
- 1 tbsp fresh dill, chopped (5g)

Instructions:

1. Preheat oven to 375°F (190°C).
2. Mix salmon, egg, almond flour, dill, onion, salt, and pepper. Form 4 patties.
3. Place on a parchment-lined baking sheet and bake for 20 minutes, flipping halfway.
4. Mix yogurt, lemon juice, and dill for the sauce. Serve cakes with a dollop on top.

Nutritional Facts (Per Serving): Calories: 350 | Carbohydrates: 8g | Protein: 22g | Fat: 14g | Sugars: 2g | Fiber: 3g | Sodium: 480mg

Glycemic Index: Salmon: Low (GI = 0) | Almond flour: Low (GI = 10) | Yogurt: Low (GI = 15)

Baked Trout with Roasted Fennel and Lemon

Prep: 10 minutes | Cook: 25 minutes | Serves: 2

Ingredients:

- 2 whole trout, gutted and cleaned (300g)
- 1 fennel bulb, sliced (150g)
- 1 lemon, sliced
- 2 tbsp olive oil (30ml)
- 1 clove garlic, minced (5g)
- Salt and pepper to taste

Instructions:

1. Preheat oven to 375°F (190°C).
2. Stuff trout with lemon slices and garlic. Place on a baking tray.
3. Toss fennel with olive oil, salt, and pepper. Arrange around fish.
4. Bake for 25 minutes until fish flakes easily. Serve warm.

Nutritional Facts (Per Serving): Calories: 350 | Carbohydrates: 9g | Protein: 22g | Fat: 14g | Sugars: 3g | Fiber: 4g | Sodium: 450mg

Glycemic Index: Trout: Low (GI = 0) | Fennel: Low (GI = 15)

Grilled Swordfish Steaks with Zucchini Ribbons

Prep: 10 minutes | Cook: 10 minutes | Serves: 2

Ingredients:

- 2 swordfish steaks (170g each)
- 2 medium zucchinis, spiralized or sliced into ribbons (300g)
- 1 tbsp olive oil (15ml)
- Juice of 1 lemon (30ml)
- 1 tsp dried oregano (2g)
- Salt and pepper to taste

Instructions:

1. Rub swordfish with half the olive oil, lemon juice, oregano, salt, and pepper.
2. Grill over medium-high heat for 4–5 minutes per side until cooked through.
3. Sauté zucchini ribbons with remaining olive oil in a skillet for 2–3 minutes until just tender.
4. Serve swordfish on top of warm zucchini ribbons.

Nutritional Facts (Per Serving): Calories: 350 | Carbohydrates: 8g | Protein: 22g | Fat: 15g | Sugars: 3g | Fiber: 4g | Sodium: 480mg

Glycemic Index: Swordfish: Low (GI = 0) | Zucchini: Low (GI = 15)

Fish Lettuce Tacos with Avocado Lime Sauce

Prep: 15 minutes | Cook: 10 minutes | Serves: 2

Ingredients:

- 6 oz white fish fillets (cod or tilapia), diced (170g)
- 1/2 avocado, mashed (75g)
- 4 large lettuce leaves (60g)
- 2 tbsp plain Greek yogurt (30g)
- Juice of 1 lime (30ml)
- 1 tbsp olive oil (15ml)
- Salt and pepper to taste

Instructions:

1. Heat olive oil in a skillet and sauté diced fish with salt and pepper for 7–8 minutes until flaky.
2. In a small bowl, mix mashed avocado, Greek yogurt, and lime juice to make the sauce.
3. Spoon fish into lettuce leaves, drizzle with avocado lime sauce, and serve immediately.

Nutritional Facts (Per Serving): Calories: 350 | Carbohydrates: 10g | Protein: 22g | Fat: 14g | Sugars: 2g | Fiber: 5g | Sodium: 460mg

Glycemic Index: White fish: Low (GI = 0) | Avocado: Low (GI = 15) | Lettuce: Low (GI = 10)

Sardine and Chickpea Salad with Lemon Mustard Dressing

Prep: 10 minutes | Cook: None | Serves: 2

Ingredients:

- 1 can sardines in olive oil, drained (120g)
- 1/2 cup cooked chickpeas (80g)
- 2 cups baby spinach (60g)
- 1 tbsp Dijon mustard (15g)
- Juice of 1 lemon (30ml)
- 1 tbsp olive oil (15ml)
- Salt and pepper to taste

Instructions:

1. In a large bowl, combine sardines, chickpeas, and spinach.
2. In a separate bowl, whisk together Dijon mustard, lemon juice, olive oil, salt, and pepper.
3. Drizzle dressing over salad and toss gently. Serve fresh.

Nutritional Facts (Per Serving): Calories: 350 | Carbohydrates: 14g | Protein: 22g | Fat: 15g | Sugars: 2g | Fiber: 5g | Sodium: 500mg

Glycemic Index: Sardines: Low (GI = 0) | Chickpeas: Low (GI = 28) | Spinach: Low (GI = 15)

Steamed Cod with Ginger-Garlic Cabbage

Prep: 10 minutes | **Cook:** 15 minutes | **Serves:** 2

Ingredients:

- 2 cod fillets (170g each)
- 2 cups shredded cabbage (150g)
- 1 tbsp grated fresh ginger (10g)
- 1 clove garlic, minced (5g)
- 1 tbsp olive oil (15ml)
- 1 tbsp lemon juice (15ml)
- Salt and pepper to taste

Instructions:

1. Steam cod fillets for 10–12 minutes until opaque and flaky.
2. Meanwhile, sauté cabbage in olive oil with garlic and ginger for 3–5 minutes until tender.
3. Drizzle lemon juice over cabbage and season with salt and pepper.
4. Serve cod on a bed of cabbage.

Nutritional Facts (Per Serving): Calories: 350 | Carbohydrates: 10g | Protein: 22g | Fat: 15g | Sugars: 3g | Fiber: 4g | Sodium: 480mg

Glycemic Index: Cod: Low (GI = 0) | Cabbage: Low (GI = 15)

Grilled Tilapia with Roasted Eggplant and Tomato

Prep: 10 minutes | **Cook:** 20 minutes | **Serves:** 2

Ingredients:

- 2 tilapia fillets (170g each)
- 1 cup eggplant, diced (150g)
- 1/2 cup cherry tomatoes, halved (100g)
- 1 tbsp olive oil (15ml)
- 1 tsp dried thyme (2g)
- Salt and pepper to taste

Instructions:

1. Preheat oven to 400°F (200°C). Toss eggplant and tomatoes with olive oil, thyme, salt, and pepper. Roast for 15–20 minutes.
2. Grill tilapia over medium heat for 4–5 minutes per side until cooked through.
3. Serve grilled tilapia with roasted vegetables on the side.

Nutritional Facts (Per Serving): Calories: 350 | Carbohydrates: 12g | Protein: 22g | Fat: 15g | Sugars: 5g | Fiber: 4g | Sodium: 480mg

Glycemic Index: Tilapia: Low (GI = 0) | Eggplant: Low (GI = 15) | Tomatoes: Low (GI = 15)

Lemon-Parsley Scallops with Sautéed Zucchini

Prep: 10 minutes | **Cook:** 10 minutes | **Serves:** 2

Ingredients:

- 10 sea scallops (200g)
- 1 medium zucchini, sliced (150g)
- 2 tbsp olive oil (30ml)
- 1 tbsp chopped fresh parsley (15g)
- Juice of 1/2 lemon (15ml)
- Salt and pepper to taste

Instructions:

1. Heat 1 tbsp olive oil in a skillet. Sear scallops for 2 minutes per side until golden. Remove and set aside.
2. In the same skillet, sauté zucchini with remaining olive oil, parsley, lemon juice, salt, and pepper for 5–6 minutes until tender.
3. Serve scallops over sautéed zucchini.

Nutritional Facts (Per Serving): Calories: 350 | Carbohydrates: 10g | Protein: 22g | Fat: 15g | Sugars: 3g | Fiber: 3g | Sodium: 470mg

Glycemic Index: Scallops: Low (GI = 0) | Zucchini: Low (GI = 15) | Lemon: Low (GI = 15)

Vegetarian and Plant-Based Options to Keep Blood Sugar Steady

Roasted Veggie Salad with Pumpkin Seeds & Lemon Vinaigrette

Prep: 10 minutes | Cook: 20 minutes | Serves: 2

Ingredients:

- 1 cup diced zucchini (150g)
- 1 cup diced bell pepper (150g)
- 1/2 cup diced red onion (75g)
- 2 tbsp olive oil (30ml)
- 2 tbsp pumpkin seeds (30g)
- Juice of 1 lemon (30ml)
- 1 tsp Dijon mustard (5g)
- Salt and pepper to taste

Instructions:

1. Preheat oven to 400°F (200°C). Roast veggies with 1 tbsp oil, salt, pepper — 20 min.
2. Whisk lemon juice, 1 tbsp oil, mustard.
3. Toss veggies with seeds, drizzle dressing. Serve warm or cooled.

Nutritional Facts (Per Serving): Calories: 350 | Sugars: 6g | Fat: 15g | Carbohydrates: 20g | Protein: 18g | Fiber: 6g | Sodium: 450mg

Glycemic Index: Zucchini: Low (GI = 15) | Bell Pepper: Low (GI = 15) | Pumpkin Seeds: Low (GI = 25)

Zoodle and Arugula Salad with Lemon-Parmesan Dressing

Prep: 10 minutes | Cook: 0 minutes | Serves: 2

Ingredients:

- 2 medium zucchinis, spiralized (300g)
- 4 cups arugula (120g)
- 2 tbsp grated Parmesan cheese (30g)
- 2 tbsp olive oil (30ml)
- Juice of 1 lemon (30ml)
- 1 tsp low carb sweetener (5g)
- Salt and pepper to taste

Instructions:

1. Whisk oil, lemon juice, Parmesan, sweetener, salt, pepper.
2. Toss zoodles & arugula.
3. Drizzle dressing. Serve.

Nutritional Facts (Per Serving): Calories: 350 | Sugars: 3g | Fat: 15g | Carbohydrates: 18g | Protein: 20g | Fiber: 6g | Sodium: 480mg

Glycemic Index: Zucchini: Low (GI = 15) | Arugula: Low (GI = 10) | Parmesan: Low (GI = 15)

Spinach and Quinoa Salad with Sunflower Seeds and Lemon Zest

Prep: 10 minutes | Cook: 15 minutes | Serves: 2

Ingredients:

- 1/2 cup cooked quinoa (90g)
- 4 cups baby spinach (120g)
- 2 tbsp sunflower seeds (30g)
- 1 tbsp olive oil (15ml)
- Juice and zest of 1/2 lemon (15ml juice)
- Salt and pepper to taste

Instructions:

1. Toss quinoa, spinach, and seeds.
2. Whisk oil, lemon juice, zest, salt, pepper.
3. Drizzle dressing, toss again. Serve.

Nutritional Facts (Per Serving): Calories: 350 | Sugars: 2g | Fat: 15g | Carbohydrates: 20g | Protein: 18g | Fiber: 5g | Sodium: 450mg

Glycemic Index: Quinoa: Medium (GI = 53) | Spinach: Low (GI = 15) | Sunflower Seeds: Low (GI = 35)

Avocado and Baby Kale Salad with Cucumber and Herb Dressing

Prep: 10 minutes | Cook: 0 minutes | Serves: 2

Ingredients:

- 1/2 avocado, diced (75g)
- 4 cups baby kale (120g)
- 1/2 cucumber, sliced (75g)
- 2 tbsp olive oil (30ml)
- 1 tbsp chopped fresh dill (15g)
- Juice of 1 lemon (30ml)
- Salt and pepper to taste

Instructions:

1. In a large bowl, toss baby kale, avocado, and cucumber together.
2. In a small bowl, whisk together olive oil, lemon juice, fresh dill, salt, and pepper.
3. Drizzle the herb dressing over the salad and toss gently. Serve fresh.

Nutritional Facts (Per Serving): Calories: 350 | Sugars: 3g | Fat: 16g | Carbohydrates: 14g | Protein: 18g | Fiber: 6g | Sodium: 400mg

Glycemic Index: Avocado: Low (GI = 15) | Kale: Low (GI = 10) | Cucumber: Low (GI = 15)

Roasted Eggplant Salad with Tahini and Pomegranate

Prep: 15 minutes | Cook: 20 minutes | Serves: 2

Ingredients:

- 1 medium eggplant, diced (200g)
- 2 tbsp olive oil (30ml)
- 1 tbsp tahini (15g)
- 2 tbsp pomegranate seeds (30g)
- 1 tbsp lemon juice (15ml)
- 1 clove garlic, minced (5g)
- Salt and pepper to taste

Instructions:

1. Preheat oven to 400°F (200°C). Toss diced eggplant with 1 tbsp olive oil, salt, and pepper. Roast for 20 minutes until tender.
2. In a small bowl, whisk together tahini, lemon juice, garlic, and the remaining olive oil.
3. Toss roasted eggplant with the tahini dressing and top with pomegranate seeds. Serve warm or at room temperature.

Nutritional Facts (Per Serving): Calories: 350 | Sugars: 6g | Fat: 14g | Carbohydrates: 20g | Protein: 18g | Fiber: 6g | Sodium: 450mg

Glycemic Index: Eggplant: Low (GI = 15) | Pomegranate Seeds: Medium (GI = 35) | Tahini: Low (GI = 40)

Eggplant Rollatini with Ricotta and Spinach

Prep: 15 minutes | Cook: 25 minutes | Serves: 2

Ingredients:

- 1 medium eggplant, thinly sliced lengthwise (200g)
- 1/2 cup ricotta cheese (120g)
- 1/2 cup cooked spinach, chopped (60g)
- 1/4 cup grated Parmesan (30g)
- 1 clove garlic, minced (5g)
- 1 tbsp olive oil (15ml)
- Salt and pepper to taste

Instructions:

1. Preheat oven to 375°F (190°C). Brush eggplant slices with olive oil, season with salt and pepper, and bake for 10 minutes until tender.
2. In a bowl, mix ricotta, spinach, Parmesan, garlic, salt, and pepper.
3. Roll the ricotta mixture inside each eggplant slice and place them in a baking dish.
4. Bake for another 15 minutes.
5. Serve warm.

Nutritional Facts (Per Serving): Calories: 350 | Sugars: 4g | Fat: 15g | Carbohydrates: 18g | Protein: 20g | Fiber: 6g | Sodium: 480mg

Glycemic Index: Eggplant: Low (GI = 15) | Ricotta: Low (GI = 15) | Spinach: Low (GI = 15)

Cauliflower Tabbouleh with Cucumber, Tomato, and Mint

Prep: 10 minutes | Cook: 0 minutes | Serves: 2

Ingredients:

- 2 cups grated cauliflower (300g)
- 1/2 cup diced cucumber (75g)
- 1/2 cup diced tomatoes (75g)
- 2 tbsp chopped fresh mint (15g)
- 2 tbsp olive oil (30ml)
- Juice of 1 lemon (30ml)
- Salt and pepper to taste

Instructions:

1. In a large bowl, combine grated cauliflower, cucumber, tomatoes, and mint.
2. In a small bowl, whisk together olive oil, lemon juice, salt, and pepper.
3. Pour the dressing over the cauliflower mixture and toss to combine. Serve chilled.

Nutritional Facts (Per Serving): Calories: 350 | Sugars: 5g | Fat: 14g | Carbohydrates: 20g | Protein: 18g | Fiber: 7g | Sodium: 400mg

Glycemic Index: Cauliflower: Low (GI = 15) | Cucumber: Low (GI = 15) | Tomatoes: Low (GI = 15)

Kale and Quinoa Stuffed Acorn Squash with Tahini Drizzle

Prep: 15 minutes | Cook: 30 minutes | Serves: 2

Ingredients:

- 1 acorn squash, halved and seeded (400g)
- 1/2 cup cooked quinoa (90g)
- 1 cup chopped kale (60g)
- 1 tbsp olive oil (15ml)
- 1 tbsp tahini (15g)
- 1 tbsp lemon juice (15ml)
- 1 clove garlic, minced (5g)
- Salt and pepper to taste

Instructions:

1. Preheat oven to 400°F (200°C). Brush acorn squash halves with olive oil, season with salt and pepper, and roast for 30 minutes until tender.
2. In a skillet, sauté kale in 1 tbsp olive oil until wilted. Mix with cooked quinoa and season with salt and pepper.
3. Stuff the roasted acorn squash halves with the quinoa-kale mixture.
4. In a small bowl, whisk together tahini, lemon juice, garlic, salt, and pepper. Drizzle over the stuffed squash. Serve warm.

Nutritional Facts (Per Serving): Calories: 350 | Sugars: 8g | Fat: 15g | Carbohydrates: 30g | Protein: 18g | Fiber: 7g | Sodium: 450mg

Glycemic Index: Acorn Squash: Medium (GI = 50) | Quinoa: Medium (GI = 53) | Kale: Low (GI = 15) | Tahini: Low (GI = 40)

Lentil and Vegetable Stew with Fresh Herbs

Prep: 10 minutes | Cook: 25 minutes | Serves: 2

Ingredients:

- 1/2 cup dried lentils (100g)
- 1/2 cup diced carrots (75g)
- 1/2 cup diced zucchini (75g)
- 1/4 cup diced onion (40g)
- 2 cups vegetable broth (480ml)
- 1 tbsp olive oil (15ml)
- 1 clove garlic, minced (5g)
- 1 tbsp fresh parsley, chopped (15g)
- Salt and pepper to taste

Instructions:

1. Heat olive oil in a large pot over medium heat. Add garlic and onion, sauté for 3 minutes.
2. Add carrots, zucchini, lentils, and vegetable broth. Bring to a boil, then reduce heat and simmer for 20-25 minutes until lentils are tender.
3. Stir in fresh parsley, season with salt and pepper, and serve warm.

Nutritional Facts (Per Serving): Calories: 350 | Sugars: 6g | Fat: 14g | Carbohydrates: 30g | Protein: 18g | Fiber: 8g | Sodium: 480mg

Glycemic Index: Lentils: Low (GI = 32) | Carrots: Medium (GI = 35) | Zucchini: Low (GI = 15)

Orange and Spinach Salad with Almonds

Prep: 10 minutes | **Cook:** 0 minutes | **Serves:** 2

Ingredients:

- 4 cups baby spinach (120g)
- 1 orange, segmented (150g)
- 2 tbsp sliced almonds (30g)
- 1 tbsp olive oil (15ml)
- 1 tbsp lemon juice (15ml)
- 1 tsp low carb sweetener (5g)
- Salt and pepper to taste

Instructions:

1. In a large bowl, toss spinach with orange segments and sliced almonds.
2. In a small bowl, whisk together olive oil, lemon juice, sweetener, salt, and pepper.
3. Drizzle the dressing over the salad and toss gently.
4. Serve fresh.

Nutritional Facts (Per Serving): Calories: 350 | Sugars: 7g | Fat: 15g | Carbohydrates: 20g | Protein: 18g | Fiber: 6g | Sodium: 400mg

Glycemic Index: Orange: Medium (GI = 43) | Spinach: Low (GI = 15) | Almonds: Low (GI = 10)

Stuffed Bell Peppers with Quinoa, Chickpeas, and Herbs

Prep: 15 minutes | **Cook:** 25 minutes | **Serves:** 2

Ingredients:

- 2 medium bell peppers, halved and seeded (300g)
- 1/2 cup cooked quinoa (90g)
- 1/2 cup canned chickpeas, rinsed and drained (90g)
- 2 tbsp chopped fresh parsley (15g)
- 1 tbsp olive oil (15ml)
- 1 tbsp lemon juice (15ml)
- Salt and pepper to taste

Instructions:

1. Preheat oven to 375°F (190°C).
2. In a bowl, mix cooked quinoa, chickpeas, parsley, lemon juice, olive oil, salt, and pepper.
3. Stuff the bell pepper halves with the mixture and place in a baking dish.
4. Bake for 20–25 minutes until peppers are tender. Serve warm.

Nutritional Facts (Per Serving): Calories: 350 | Carbohydrates: 25g | Protein: 18g | Fat: 14g | Fiber: 7g | Sugars: 5g | Sodium: 480mg

Glycemic Index: Bell pepper: Low (GI = 15) | Quinoa: Medium (GI = 53) | Chickpeas: Low (GI = 28)

Chickpea and Kale Stir-Fry with Garlic and Lemon

Prep: 10 minutes | **Cook:** 10 minutes | **Serves:** 2

Ingredients:

- 1 cup canned chickpeas, rinsed and drained (170g)
- 3 cups chopped kale (90g)
- 1 clove garlic, minced (5g)
- 1 tbsp olive oil (15ml)
- Juice of 1/2 lemon (15ml)
- Salt and pepper to taste

Instructions:

1. Heat olive oil in a pan over medium heat. Add garlic and cook for 1 minute.
2. Add chickpeas and cook for 3–4 minutes until lightly golden.
3. Stir in kale and sauté until wilted, about 3 minutes. Add lemon juice, salt, and pepper.
4. Serve warm.

Nutritional Facts (Per Serving): Calories: 350 | Carbohydrates: 24g | Protein: 18g | Fat: 14g | Fiber: 6g | Sugars: 3g | Sodium: 450mg

Glycemic Index: Chickpeas: Low (GI = 28) | Kale: Low (GI = 10)

Sweet Potato and Black Bean Salad with Lime-Cilantro Dressing

Prep: 15 minutes | Cook: 15 minutes | Serves: 2

Ingredients:

- 1 small sweet potato, peeled and diced (150g)
- 1/2 cup canned black beans, rinsed and drained (90g)
- 1/4 cup diced red onion (40g)
- 2 tbsp chopped fresh cilantro (10g)
- 1 tbsp olive oil (15ml)
- Juice of 1 lime (30ml)
- Salt and pepper to taste

Instructions:

1. Boil or steam sweet potato for 10–12 minutes until tender. Let cool slightly.
2. In a bowl, combine sweet potato, black beans, red onion, and cilantro.
3. In a small bowl, whisk olive oil, lime juice, salt, and pepper. Toss with the salad.
4. Serve warm or chilled.

Nutritional Facts (Per Serving): Calories: 350 | Carbohydrates: 30g | Protein: 18g | Fat: 14g | Fiber: 7g | Sugars: 6g | Sodium: 460mg

Glycemic Index: Sweet potato: Medium (GI = 54) | Black beans: Low (GI = 30)

Grilled Tofu with Sesame-Ginger Dressing and Broccoli

Prep: 10 minutes | Cook: 15 minutes | Serves: 2

Ingredients:

- 6 oz firm tofu, pressed and sliced (170g)
- 2 cups broccoli florets (200g)
- 1 tbsp sesame oil (15ml)
- 1 tbsp rice vinegar (15ml)
- 1 tsp grated fresh ginger (5g)
- 1 tsp low carb sweetener (5g)
- Salt and pepper to taste

Instructions:

1. Grill tofu slices for 3–4 minutes per side until golden.
2. Steam broccoli until just tender, about 5 minutes.
3. In a bowl, whisk sesame oil, rice vinegar, ginger, sweetener, salt, and pepper.
4. Serve grilled tofu with broccoli, drizzled with sesame-ginger dressing.

Nutritional Facts (Per Serving): Calories: 350 | Carbohydrates: 14g | Protein: 20g | Fat: 14g | Fiber: 5g | Sugars: 3g | Sodium: 460mg

Glycemic Index: Tofu: Low (GI = 15) | Broccoli: Low (GI = 15) | Sesame oil: GI = 0

Spaghetti Squash Bowl with Roasted Chickpeas and Spinach

Prep: 15 minutes | Cook: 30 minutes | Serves: 2

Ingredients:

- 1 small spaghetti squash (600g)
- 1/2 cup canned chickpeas, rinsed and drained (90g)
- 2 cups baby spinach (60g)
- 1 tbsp olive oil (15ml)
- 1 tsp smoked paprika (2g)
- Salt and pepper to taste

Instructions:

1. Preheat oven to 400°F (200°C). Cut spaghetti squash in half, remove seeds, and roast for 30 minutes.
2. Meanwhile, toss chickpeas with olive oil, paprika, salt, and pepper. Roast on a separate tray for 20 minutes.
3. Scrape squash strands into a bowl, add spinach and roasted chickpeas. Toss to combine and serve warm.

Nutritional Facts (Per Serving): Calories: 350 | Carbohydrates: 25g | Protein: 18g | Fat: 14g | Fiber: 6g | Sugars: 5g | Sodium: 470mg

Glycemic Index: Spaghetti squash: Low (GI = 41) | Chickpeas: Low (GI = 28) | Spinach: Low (GI = 15)

Lentil and Sweet Potato Patties with Herb Yogurt Sauce

Prep: 15 minutes | Cook: 20 minutes | Serves: 2

Ingredients:

- 1/2 cup cooked lentils (100g)
- 1/2 cup mashed sweet potato (100g)
- 2 tbsp oat flour (20g)
- 1/2 tsp cumin (1g)
- 1 tbsp olive oil (15ml)
- Salt and pepper to taste
- 1/4 cup plain Greek yogurt (60g)
- 1 tbsp chopped parsley (5g)
- 1 tsp lemon juice (5ml)

Instructions:

1. Mix lentils, mashed sweet potato, oat flour, cumin, salt, and pepper. Form into small patties.
2. Heat olive oil in a pan and cook patties for 4–5 minutes per side until golden.
3. In a small bowl, mix yogurt, parsley, and lemon juice to make the sauce.
4. Serve patties with a spoonful of herb yogurt sauce.

Nutritional Facts (Per Serving): Calories: 350 | Carbohydrates: 28g | Protein: 18g | Fat: 14g | Fiber: 7g | Sugars: 5g | Sodium: 460mg

Glycemic Index: Lentils: Low (GI = 32) | Sweet Potato: Medium (GI = 54) | Oat flour: Low (GI = 44)

Stuffed Bell Peppers with Black Beans and Cauliflower Rice

Prep: 15 minutes | Cook: 25 minutes | Serves: 2

Ingredients:

- 2 large bell peppers, halved and seeded (300g)
- 1/2 cup black beans, rinsed and drained (90g)
- 1 cup cauliflower rice (150g)
- 1 tbsp olive oil (15ml)
- 1/2 tsp ground cumin (1g)
- 2 tbsp chopped cilantro (10g)
- Salt and pepper to taste

Instructions:

1. Preheat oven to 375°F (190°C). Lightly oil a baking dish.
2. In a skillet, heat olive oil over medium heat. Sauté cauliflower rice with cumin, salt, and pepper for 5 minutes.
3. Stir in black beans and chopped cilantro.
4. Fill each bell pepper half with the mixture and place in the baking dish.
5. Bake for 20 minutes. Serve warm.

Nutritional Facts (Per Serving): Calories: 350 | Carbohydrates: 26g | Protein: 18g | Fat: 14g | Fiber: 8g | Sugars: 5g | Sodium: 480mg

Glycemic Index: Bell Pepper: Low (GI = 15) | Black Beans: Low (GI = 30) | Cauliflower: Low (GI = 15)

Roasted Carrot and Lentil Salad with Lemon-Cumin Dressing

Prep: 10 minutes | Cook: 25 minutes | Serves: 2

Ingredients:

- 1 cup carrots, sliced (150g)
- 1/2 cup cooked green lentils (100g)
- 2 cups arugula (60g)
- 1 tbsp olive oil (15ml)
- 1 tbsp lemon juice (15ml)
- 1/2 tsp ground cumin (1g)
- Salt and pepper to taste

Instructions:

1. Preheat oven to 400°F (200°C). Toss sliced carrots with 1/2 tbsp olive oil, salt, and pepper. Roast for 20–25 minutes until golden.
2. In a bowl, whisk the remaining olive oil with lemon juice and cumin.
3. Toss arugula, lentils, and roasted carrots in a bowl. Drizzle with dressing and serve.

Nutritional Facts (Per Serving): Calories: 350 | Carbohydrates: 27g | Protein: 18g | Fat: 14g | Fiber: 7g | Sugars: 6g | Sodium: 450mg

Glycemic Index: Carrots: Medium (GI = 35) | Lentils: Low (GI = 32) | Arugula: Low (GI = 10

Festive Dishes for Special Occasions

Seafood Paella with Brown Rice

Prep: 15 minutes | Cook: 25 minutes | Serves: 2

Ingredients:

- 1/2 cup uncooked brown rice (90g)
- 4 oz shrimp, peeled and deveined (120g)
- 4 oz mussels, cleaned (120g)
- 1/2 cup diced bell peppers (75g)
- 1/2 cup diced tomatoes (75g)
- 1/4 cup frozen peas (40g)
- 1 tbsp olive oil (15ml)
- 1 clove garlic, minced (5g)
- 1 tsp smoked paprika (5g)
- 1/4 tsp saffron (optional)
- Salt and pepper to taste

Instructions:

1. Cook rice.
2. Sauté garlic, peppers, tomatoes (5 min).
3. Add seafood, paprika, saffron, salt, pepper. Cook 5–7 min.
4. Stir in rice & peas. Heat 2–3 min. Serve.

Nutritional Facts (Per Serving): Calories: 350 | Sugars: 5g | Fat: 15g | Carbohydrates: 28g | Protein: 20g | Fiber: 6g | Sodium: 480mg

Glycemic Index: Brown rice: Medium (GI = 50) | Shrimp: Low (GI = 0) | Mussels: Low (GI = 0) | Bell Peppers: Low (GI = 15)

Herb-Roasted Whole Chicken with Garlic and Lemon

Prep: 15 minutes | Cook: 1 hour 20 minutes | Serves: 4

Ingredients:

- 1 whole chicken (3.5 lbs) (1.6kg)
- 2 tbsp olive oil (30ml)
- 1 lemon, quartered (120g)
- 4 cloves garlic, minced (20g)
- 1 tbsp fresh rosemary, chopped (15g)
- 1 tbsp fresh thyme, chopped (15g)
- Salt and pepper to taste

Instructions:

1. Preheat the oven to 375°F (190°C).
2. Rub the chicken with olive oil, minced garlic, rosemary, thyme, salt, and pepper. Stuff the cavity with lemon quarters.
3. Roast the chicken for 1 hour 20 minutes or until the internal temperature reaches 165°F (75°C). Let rest for 10 minutes before carving.

Nutritional Facts (Per Serving): Calories: 350 | Sugars: 0g | Fat: 16g | Carbohydrates: 4g | Protein: 22g | Fiber: 1g | Sodium: 550mg

Glycemic Index: Chicken: Low (GI = 0) | Lemon: Low (GI = 15)

Roast Duck with Apples and Cinnamon

Prep: 10 minutes | Cook: 1 hour 30 minutes | Serves: 4

Ingredients:

- 1 whole duck (3.5 lbs) (1.6kg)
- 2 apples, sliced (200g)
- 1 tbsp cinnamon (8g)
- 2 tbsp olive oil (30ml)
- 1 tbsp fresh thyme, chopped (15g)
- Salt and pepper to taste

Instructions:

1. Preheat the oven to 375°F (190°C).
2. Rub the duck with olive oil, cinnamon, thyme, salt, and pepper.
3. Stuff the cavity with apple slices and roast for 1 hour 30 minutes until the internal temperature reaches 165°F (75°C). Let rest for 10 minutes before carving.

Nutritional Facts (Per Serving): Calories: 350 | Sugars: 6g | Fat: 16g | Carbohydrates: 10g | Protein: 20g | Fiber: 2g | Sodium: 480mg

Glycemic Index: Duck: Low (GI = 0) | Apples: Medium (GI = 38)

Roast Turkey with Herb-Cauliflower Stuffing and Roasted Vegetables

Prep: 20 minutes | Cook: 1 hour 30 minutes | Serves: 4

Ingredients:

- 2 turkey breasts (12 oz each) (340g each)
- 2 cups cauliflower, riced (300g)
- 1 cup diced carrots (120g)
- 1 cup diced zucchini (120g)
- 2 tbsp olive oil (30ml)
- 1 tbsp fresh parsley, chopped (15g)
- 1 tbsp fresh rosemary, chopped (15g)
- Salt and pepper to taste

Instructions:

1. Preheat the oven to 375°F (190°C).
2. Toss riced cauliflower, carrots, and zucchini with olive oil, parsley, rosemary, salt, and pepper.
3. Stuff the turkey breasts with the cauliflower mixture and place in a roasting pan with the remaining vegetables. Roast for 1 hour 30 minutes or until the internal temperature reaches 165°F (75°C).

Nutritional Facts (Per Serving): Calories: 350 | Sugars: 5g | Fat: 14g | Carbohydrates: 18g | Protein: 22g | Fiber: 6g | Sodium: 500mg

Glycemic Index: Turkey: Low (GI = 0) | Cauliflower: Low (GI = 15) | Carrots: Medium (GI = 35) | Zucchini: Low (GI = 15)

Beef Wellington with Almond Flour Crust and Roasted Asparagus

Prep: 20 minutes | Cook: 30 minutes | Serves: 2

Ingredients:

- 2 beef tenderloin steaks (5 oz each) (140g each)
- 1/2 cup almond flour (50g)
- 1 tbsp butter (15g)
- 1/2 cup mushrooms, finely chopped (75g)
- 1 tbsp Dijon mustard (15g)
- 1 egg, beaten (50g)
- 8 asparagus spears (150g)
- 1 tbsp olive oil (15ml)
- Salt and pepper to taste

Instructions:

1. Preheat oven to 400°F (200°C). Sauté mushrooms in butter for 5 minutes until softened.
2. Season steaks with salt, pepper, and mustard. Wrap each steak in almond flour dough, sealing edges with beaten egg.
3. Roast asparagus with olive oil, salt, and pepper for 15-20 minutes.
4. Bake the wrapped beef for 15-20 minutes until the crust is golden and the meat is cooked to your liking.
5 Serve with roasted asparagus.

Nutritional Facts (Per Serving): Calories: 350 | Sugars: 2g | Fat: 15g | Carbohydrates: 12g | Protein: 22g | Fiber: 4g | Sodium: 480mg

Glycemic Index: Beef: Low (GI = 0) | Almond flour: Low (GI = 10) | Asparagus: Low (GI = 15)

Stuffed Turkey Roulade with Cranberry and Almond Filling

Prep: 15 minutes | Cook: 30 minutes | Serves: 2

Ingredients:

- 2 turkey breasts, thinly sliced (5 oz each) (140g each)
- 1/4 cup dried cranberries (30g)
- 2 tbsp chopped almonds (30g)
- 1 tbsp olive oil (15ml)
- 1 tbsp fresh rosemary, chopped (15g)
- 1 clove garlic, minced (5g)
- Salt and pepper to taste

Instructions:

1. Preheat oven to 375°F (190°C). Flatten turkey breasts and season with salt and pepper.
2. In a bowl, mix cranberries, almonds, rosemary, and garlic.
3 Spread the mixture on each turkey breast and roll them up.
4. Secure with toothpicks and brush with olive oil. Roast for 25-30 minutes until fully cooked.

Nutritional Facts (Per Serving): Calories: 350 | Sugars: 6g | Fat: 14g | Carbohydrates: 16g | Protein: 22g | Fiber: 4g | Sodium: 460mg

Glycemic Index: Turkey: Low (GI = 0) | Cranberries: Medium (GI = 45) | Almonds: Low (GI = 10)

Spinach & Feta Stuffed Chicken

Prep: 15 minutes | Cook: 25 minutes | Serves: 2

Ingredients:

- 2 chicken breasts (5 oz each) (140g each)
- 1/2 cup cooked spinach, chopped (60g)
- 1/4 cup crumbled feta cheese (30g)
- 2 tbsp chopped sun-dried tomatoes (30g)
- 1 tbsp olive oil (15ml)
- Salt and pepper to taste

Instructions:

1. Preheat oven to 375°F (190°C). Slice chicken breasts lengthwise to create a pocket.
2. In a bowl, mix spinach, feta, and sun-dried tomatoes. Stuff the mixture into each chicken breast and secure with toothpicks.
3. Brush with olive oil, season with salt and pepper, and bake for 25 minutes until the chicken is fully cooked.

Nutritional Facts (Per Serving): Calories: 350 | Sugars: 4g | Fat: 15g | Carbohydrates: 8g | Protein: 22g | Fiber: 3g | Sodium: 500mg

Glycemic Index: Chicken: Low (GI = 0) | Spinach: Low (GI = 15) | Feta: Low (GI = 15) | Sun-Dried Tomatoes: Medium (GI = 35)

Stuffed Pork Tenderloin with Spinach, Walnuts, and Goat Cheese

Prep: 15 minutes | Cook: 30 minutes | Serves: 2

Ingredients:

- 1 pork tenderloin (10 oz) (280g)
- 1/2 cup cooked spinach, chopped (60g)
- 2 tbsp chopped walnuts (30g)
- 1/4 cup crumbled goat cheese (30g)
- 1 tbsp olive oil (15ml)
- 1 clove garlic, minced (5g)
- Salt and pepper to taste

Instructions:

1. Preheat oven to 375°F (190°C). Butterfly the pork tenderloin and season with salt and pepper.
2. In a bowl, mix spinach, walnuts, goat cheese, and garlic. Stuff the mixture into the pork and tie it with kitchen twine.
3. Heat olive oil in a skillet and sear the pork on all sides for 5 minutes. Transfer to the oven and roast for 20-25 minutes until the internal temperature reaches 145°F (63°C).

Nutritional Facts (Per Serving): Calories: 350 | Sugars: 2g | Fat: 17g | Carbohydrates: 6g | Protein: 22g | Fiber: 2g | Sodium: 450mg

Glycemic Index: Pork: Low (GI = 0) | Spinach: Low (GI = 15) | Walnuts: Low (GI = 10)

Shepherd's Pie with Cauliflower Mash

Prep: 20 minutes | Cook: 30 minutes | Serves: 2

Ingredients:

- 1/2 lb ground beef (225g)
- 2 cups cauliflower florets (300g)
- 1/2 cup diced carrots (75g)
- 1/4 cup diced onion (40g)
- 1 tbsp olive oil (15ml)
- 1 tbsp butter (15g)
- 1/4 cup beef broth (60ml)
- Salt and pepper to taste

Instructions:

1. Preheat oven to 375°F (190°C). Boil cauliflower until tender, then mash with butter, salt, and pepper.
2. Heat olive oil in a skillet and sauté onions, carrots, and ground beef until cooked through. Add beef broth and simmer for 5 minutes.
3. Transfer the beef mixture to a baking dish, top with cauliflower mash, and bake for 20 minutes until golden.

Nutritional Facts (Per Serving): Calories: 350 | Sugars: 4g | Fat: 17g | Carbohydrates: 10g | Protein: 22g | Fiber: 4g | Sodium: 500mg

Glycemic Index: Cauliflower: Low (GI = 15) | Ground Beef: Low (GI = 0)

Stuffed Bell Peppers with Ground Turkey and Quinoa

Prep: 15 minutes | Cook: 30 minutes | Serves: 2

Ingredients:

- 2 large bell peppers, halved and deseeded (300g)
- 6 oz ground turkey (170g)
- 1/2 cup cooked quinoa (90g)
- 1/4 cup diced tomatoes (60g)
- 1 clove garlic, minced (5g)
- 1 tbsp chopped parsley (15g)
- Salt and pepper to taste
- 1 tbsp olive oil (15ml)

Instructions:

1. Preheat oven to 375°F (190°C).
2. Heat olive oil in a skillet, sauté garlic, then add turkey and cook for 6–7 minutes.
3. Stir in cooked quinoa, tomatoes, parsley, salt, and pepper.
4. Fill pepper halves with the turkey mixture, place in a baking dish, and cover with foil.
5. Bake for 25–30 minutes. Serve warm.

Nutritional Facts (Per Serving): Calories: 350 | Carbohydrates: 26g | Protein: 22g | Fat: 14g | Fiber: 6g | Sugar: 5g | Sodium: 480mg

Glycemic Index: Bell Pepper: Low (GI = 15) | Quinoa: Medium (GI = 53) | Turkey: Low (GI = 0)

Walnut-Crusted Chicken with Garlic Green Beans

Prep: 10 minutes | Cook: 25 minutes | Serves: 2

Ingredients:

- 2 chicken breasts (5 oz each) (140g each)
- 1/4 cup finely chopped walnuts (30g)
- 1 tbsp Dijon mustard (15g)
- 1 tbsp olive oil (15ml)
- Salt and pepper to taste
- 1 clove garlic, minced (5g)
- 2 cups green beans, trimmed (200g)

Instructions:

1. Preheat oven to 375°F (190°C). Brush chicken with Dijon mustard and press into chopped walnuts.
2. Place on a baking sheet and roast for 20–25 minutes until cooked through.
3. Meanwhile, sauté green beans in olive oil with garlic, salt, and pepper for 5–7 minutes.
4. Serve walnut-crusted chicken with garlic green beans.

Nutritional Facts (Per Serving): Calories: 350 | Carbohydrates: 10g | Protein: 22g | Fat: 17g | Fiber: 4g | Sugar: 2g | Sodium: 460mg

Glycemic Index: Chicken: Low (GI = 0) | Walnuts: Low (GI = 10) | Green Beans: Low (GI = 15)

Cauliflower Gratin with Almond Milk and Gruyère

Prep: 10 minutes | Cook: 25 minutes | Serves: 2

Ingredients:

- 3 cups cauliflower florets (300g)
- 1/2 cup unsweetened almond milk (120ml)
- 1/4 cup grated Gruyère cheese (30g)
- 1 tbsp almond flour (10g)
- 1 tbsp olive oil (15ml)
- Salt, pepper, and a pinch of nutmeg

Instructions:

1. Preheat oven to 375°F (190°C). Steam cauliflower until just tender, about 5 minutes.
2. In a small saucepan, warm almond milk, olive oil, nutmeg, salt, and pepper. Stir in almond flour until slightly thickened.
3. Place cauliflower in a baking dish, pour sauce over, and top with cheese.
4. Bake for 15–20 minutes until bubbly and golden.

Nutritional Facts (Per Serving): Calories: 350 | Carbohydrates: 12g | Protein: 18g | Fat: 17g | Fiber: 5g | Sugar: 3g | Sodium: 450mg

Glycemic Index: Cauliflower: Low (GI = 15) | Almond Milk: Low (GI = 30) | Gruyère: Low (GI = 0)

Beef and Mushroom Skillet with Rosemary

Prep: 10 minutes | Cook: 20 minutes | Serves: 2

Ingredients:

- 6 oz lean beef, sliced (170g)
- 1 cup mushrooms, sliced (150g)
- 1 small onion, chopped (70g)
- Salt and pepper to taste
- 1 tsp chopped rosemary (2g)
- 1 tbsp olive oil (15ml)

Instructions:

1. Heat oil in a skillet over medium heat.
2. Sauté onion and mushrooms for 5 minutes. Add beef and rosemary, cook 8–10 minutes.
3. Season with salt and pepper. Serve hot.

Nutritional Facts (Per Serving): Calories: 350 | Carbs: 10g | Protein: 22g | Fat: 16g | Sugar: 4g | Fiber: 3g | Sodium: 460mg

Glycemic Index: Beef: Low (GI = 0) | Mushrooms: Low (GI = 15) | Onion: Low (GI = 10)

Stuffed Acorn Squash with Wild Rice and Cranberries

Prep: 15 minutes | Cook: 30 minutes | Serves: 2

Ingredients:

- 1 small acorn squash, halved (400g)
- 1/2 cup cooked wild rice (90g)
- 2 tbsp dried cranberries (20g)
- 1/2 tsp cinnamon (1g)
- 1 tbsp olive oil (15ml)
- 2 tbsp chopped pecans (20g)
- Salt and pepper to taste

Instructions:

1. Preheat oven to 400°F (200°C). Brush squash with oil, roast 30 minutes.
2. Mix wild rice, cranberries, pecans, cinnamon, salt, and pepper.
3. Stuff squash halves and serve warm.

Nutritional Facts (Per Serving): Calories: 350 | Carbs: 30g | Protein: 18g | Fat: 14g | Sugar: 7g | Fiber: 6g | Sodium: 450mg

Glycemic Index: Acorn Squash: Medium (GI = 50) | Wild Rice: Medium (GI = 45) | Cranberries: Medium (GI = 45)

Salmon Fillet with Pomegranate Glaze and Herbs

Prep: 10 minutes | Cook: 15 minutes | Serves: 2

Ingredients:

- 2 salmon fillets (6 oz each) (170g each)
- 2 tbsp pomegranate juice (30ml)
- 1 tsp low carb sweetener (5g)
- 1 tbsp chopped parsley (5g)
- 1 tbsp olive oil (15ml)
- Salt and pepper to taste

Instructions:

1. Preheat oven to 375°F (190°C).
2. Sear salmon in oil for 2–3 min. In bowl, mix juice, sweetener, salt, pepper.
3. Glaze salmon, transfer to oven for 10 min. Top with parsley.

Nutritional Facts (Per Serving): Calories: 350 | Carbs: 8g | Protein: 22g | Fat: 15g | Sugar: 3g | Fiber: 2g | Sodium: 440mg

Glycemic Index: Salmon: Low (GI = 0) | Pomegranate: Medium (GI = 53)

Zucchini Rollatini with Ricotta and Walnut Filling

Prep: 15 minutes | Cook: 20 minutes | Serves: 2

Ingredients:

- 2 medium zucchinis, sliced thin lengthwise (300g)
- 1/2 cup ricotta cheese (120g)
- 2 tbsp chopped walnuts (20g)
- 1 tbsp olive oil (15ml)
- 1 tsp dried oregano (2g)
- Salt and pepper to taste

Instructions:

1. Preheat oven to 375°F (190°C). Brush zucchini slices with oil and bake 5–7 minutes.
2. Mix ricotta, walnuts, oregano, salt, and pepper.
3. Roll mixture into zucchini slices. Place in dish and bake for 10–12 minutes.

Nutritional Facts (Per Serving): Calories: 350 | Carbs: 10g | Protein: 18g | Fat: 16g | Sugar: 4g | Fiber: 4g | Sodium: 450mg

Glycemic Index: Zucchini: Low (GI = 15) | Ricotta: Low (GI = 15) | Walnuts: Low (GI = 10)

Stuffed Bell Peppers with Lentils and Herbs

Prep: 15 minutes | Cook: 25 minutes | Serves: 2

Ingredients:

- 2 bell peppers, halved and seeded (200g)
- 1/2 cup cooked lentils (100g)
- 1/4 cup diced tomatoes (60g)
- 2 tbsp chopped parsley (10g)
- 1 tbsp olive oil (15ml)
- Salt and pepper to taste

Instructions:

1. Preheat oven to 375°F (190°C).
2. In a bowl, mix lentils, tomatoes, parsley, oil, salt, and pepper.
3. Stuff the peppers and bake for 25 minutes. Serve warm.

Nutritional Facts (Per Serving): Calories: 350 | Carbs: 28g | Protein: 20g | Fat: 14g | Sugar: 5g | Fiber: 7g | Sodium: 460mg

Glycemic Index: Bell Peppers: Low (GI = 15) | Lentils: Low (GI = 32) | Tomatoes: Low (GI = 15)

Grilled Eggplant Steaks with Herbed Yogurt Sauce

Prep: 10 minutes | Cook: 15 minutes | Serves: 2

Ingredients:

- 2 eggplant slices, 1-inch thick (300g)
- 1/2 cup plain Greek yogurt (120g)
- 1 tbsp chopped mint (5g)
- 1 tbsp lemon juice (15ml)
- 1 tbsp olive oil (15ml)
- Salt and pepper to taste

Instructions:

1. Brush eggplant slices with oil, salt, and pepper. Grill 6–7 minutes per side.
2. Mix yogurt, mint, lemon juice, salt, and pepper for sauce.
3. Serve eggplant steaks with herbed yogurt on top.

Nutritional Facts (Per Serving): Calories: 350 | Carbs: 12g | Protein: 22g | Fat: 14g | Sugar: 5g | Fiber: 5g | Sodium: 480mg

Glycemic Index: Eggplant: Low (GI = 15) | Greek Yogurt: Low (GI = 15)

CHAPTER 7: BONUSES AND USEFUL MATERIALS

60-Day Grocery Shopping Templates for Diabetes

To make your journey easier, we've prepared these 60-day grocery shopping templates tailored specifically for individuals managing diabetes. With these ingredients, you can prepare the specified meals for the specified days. Adjust quantities based on your specific dietary needs and preferences.

Ensure to choose fresh, unprocessed items and always check labels for added sugars and preservatives. Planning meals with these whole foods will support a balanced and nutritious diabetic-friendly diet.

Happy cooking and healthy eating

Grocery Shopping List for 7-Day Meal Plan

Meat & Poultry

Ground turkey – 400 g / 14 oz (Turkey Sausage and Veggie Scramble, Stuffed Bell Peppers with Ground Turkey and Zucchini, Garlic Turkey Meatball Soup with Greens)
Chicken breast – 200 g / 7 oz (Quinoa Bowl with Grilled Chicken and Roasted Peppers)
Turkey sausage – 150 g / 5 oz (Turkey Sausage and Veggie Scramble)
Turkey breast, sliced or cubed – 150 g / 5 oz (Turkey and Cheese Skewers with Olives)
Lean beef stew meat – 250 g / 9 oz (Beef and Vegetable Stew with Carrots and Celery)

Fish & Seafood

Fresh tilapia fillets – 180 g / 6 oz (Grilled Tilapia with Roasted Eggplant and Tomato)
Raw shrimp, peeled and deveined – 150 g / 5 oz (Grilled Shrimp and Asparagus Salad with Garlic-Lemon Dressing)
Swordfish steaks – 180 g / 6 oz (Grilled Swordfish Steaks with Zucchini Ribbons)

Vegetables

Bell peppers (red, yellow, green) – 6 large (Stuffed Bell Peppers with Ground Turkey and Zucchini, Egg-Stuffed Bell Pepper Boats, Grilled Chicken and Roasted Peppers, Zoodle and Arugula Salad)
Carrots – 3 medium (Beef and Vegetable Stew with Carrots and Celery)
Celery stalks – 5 large (Beef and Vegetable Stew with Carrots and Celery, Celery Sticks with Almond Butter and Chia Seeds)
Cucumber – 3 medium (Cucumber Slices with Avocado and Hummus, Cottage Cheese with Sliced Tomatoes and Cucumber)
Spinach – 200 g / 7 oz (Kale and Spinach Salad with Balsamic Vinaigrette and Feta, Low-Carb Cottage Cheese and Spinach Pancakes, Kale and Coconut Protein Bowl)
Kale – 250 g / 9 oz (Kale and Spinach Salad with Balsamic Vinaigrette and Feta, Kale and Coconut Protein Bowl, Spelt Bowl with Sautéed Kale and Poached Egg)
Zucchini – 4 medium (Stuffed Bell Peppers with Ground Turkey and Zucchini, Grilled Swordfish Steaks with Zucchini Ribbons)
Eggplant – 2 large (Grilled Tilapia with Roasted Eggplant and Tomato)

Tomatoes – 5 medium (Grilled Tilapia with Roasted Eggplant and Tomato, Cottage Cheese with Sliced Tomatoes and Cucumber)
Baby kale – 100 g / 3.5 oz (Barley and Mushroom Bowl with Baby Kale)
Arugula – 60 g / 2 oz (Zoodle and Arugula Salad with Lemon-Parmesan Dressing)
Asparagus – 1 bunch (about 250 g / 9 oz) (Grilled Shrimp and Asparagus Salad with Garlic-Lemon Dressing)
Red cabbage – 1/4 head (about 200 g / 7 oz) (Barley Bowl with Grilled Tofu and Red Cabbage)
Cauliflower – 1 medium head (about 700 g / 25 oz) (Cauliflower Rice Stir-Fry with Scrambled Eggs and Garlic, Cauliflower Tabbouleh with Mint and Lemon Vinaigrette)
Garlic – 2 bulbs (Creamy Mushroom Soup with Roasted Garlic and Herbs, Cauliflower Rice Stir-Fry, Grilled Shrimp and Asparagus Salad)
Mushrooms (button or cremini) – 300 g / 10 oz (Creamy Mushroom Soup with Roasted Garlic and Herbs, Barley and Mushroom Bowl with Baby Kale)
Mint, fresh – 1 small bunch (Cauliflower Tabbouleh with Mint and Lemon Vinaigrette)
Lemon – 4 medium (Kale and Spinach Salad, Zoodle and Arugula Salad, Cauliflower Tabbouleh, Grilled Shrimp Salad)
Mixed salad greens – 1 small bag (about 100 g / 3.5 oz) (Salads & Bowls, extra as needed)

Fruits

Avocado – 3 large (Cucumber Slices with Avocado and Hummus, Zoodle and Arugula Salad)
Blueberries – 120 g / 1 cup (Almond Butter Couscous Porridge with Blueberries and Flaxseeds, Coconut Yogurt Parfait with Berries and Seeds)
Raspberries – 120 g / 1 cup (Sugar-Free Raspberry Mousse with Whipped Coconut Cream)
Mixed berries (blueberries, strawberries, blackberries) – 180 g / 1.5 cups (Coconut Yogurt Parfait with Berries and Seeds)
Lemon (already listed under Vegetables)

Grains & Bread

Couscous, whole wheat – 70 g / 1/2 cup dry (Almond Butter Couscous Porridge with Blueberries and Flaxseeds)
Quinoa, dry – 80 g / 1/2 cup (Quinoa Bowl with Grilled Chicken and Roasted Peppers)
Barley, pearl – 100 g / 2/3 cup dry (Barley Bowl with Grilled Tofu and Red Cabbage, Barley and Mushroom Bowl with Baby Kale)
Spelt grain, dry – 70 g / 1/2 cup (Spelt Bowl with Sautéed Kale and Poached Egg)
Tofu, firm – 150 g / 5 oz (Barley Bowl with Grilled Tofu and Red Cabbage)

Dairy & Eggs

Eggs – 14 large (Egg-Stuffed Bell Pepper Boats, Cauliflower Rice Stir-Fry with Scrambled Eggs and Garlic, Spelt Bowl with Sautéed Kale and Poached Egg, Low-Carb Cottage Cheese and Spinach Pancakes)
Cottage cheese, low-fat – 250 g / 1 cup (Low-Carb Cottage Cheese and Spinach Pancakes, Cottage Cheese with Sliced Tomatoes and Cucumber, Turkey and Cheese Skewers with Olives)
Feta cheese – 100 g / 3.5 oz (Kale and Spinach Salad with Balsamic Vinaigrette and Feta)
Parmesan cheese – 50 g / 2 oz (Zoodle and Arugula Salad with Lemon-Parmesan Dressing)
Coconut yogurt, unsweetened – 150 g / 2/3 cup (Coconut Yogurt Parfait with Berries and Seeds)
Coconut cream – 100 ml / 6 tbsp (Keto Pumpkin Pie Bites with Coconut Cream, Sugar-Free Raspberry Mousse with Whipped Coconut Cream)
Hard cheese (like cheddar or gouda) – 60 g / 2 oz (Turkey and Cheese Skewers with Olives)

Nuts, Seeds & Nut Butter

Almond butter – 6 tbsp / 90 g (Almond Butter Couscous Porridge with Blueberries and Flaxseeds, Celery Sticks with Almond Butter and Chia Seeds)
Chia seeds – 6 tbsp / 60 g (Celery Sticks with Almond Butter and Chia Seeds, Cinnamon Vanilla Chia Custard, Coconut Yogurt Parfait)
Flaxseeds, ground – 3 tbsp / 30 g (Almond Butter Couscous Porridge with Blueberries and Flaxseeds)

Pumpkin seeds – 2 tbsp / 20 g (Coconut Yogurt Parfait with Berries and Seeds)
Mixed nuts (almonds, walnuts) – 40 g / 1/3 cup (Snacks/Optional, Cinnamon Vanilla Chia Custard)

Pantry Staples

Extra virgin olive oil – 120 ml / 1/2 cup (Kale and Spinach Salad, Grilled Dishes, Stir-Fries, Cauliflower Tabbouleh)
 Coconut oil – 2 tbsp / 30 ml (Keto Pumpkin Pie Bites with Coconut Cream)
 Hummus – 100 g / 1/3 cup (Cucumber Slices with Avocado and Hummus)
 Cinnamon, ground – 2 tsp (Cinnamon Vanilla Chia Custard)
 Vanilla extract – 2 tsp (Cinnamon Vanilla Chia Custard, Sugar-Free Raspberry Mousse)
 Pumpkin purée, unsweetened – 100 g / 1/2 cup (Keto Pumpkin Pie Bites with Coconut Cream)
 Dijon mustard – 1 tbsp / 15 ml (Kale and Spinach Salad, Lemon-Parmesan Dressing)
 White wine vinegar or apple cider vinegar – 3 tbsp / 45 ml (Salads, Vinaigrettes)
 Tahini – 2 tbsp / 30 g (Cauliflower Tabbouleh with Mint and Lemon Vinaigrette)
 Dried herbs: oregano, thyme, rosemary – 1 tsp each (Mediterranean stews, Roasted Veg, Soups)
 Salt and black pepper – to taste (General use)
 Baking powder – 1 tsp (Low-Carb Cottage Cheese and Spinach Pancakes)

Grocery Shopping List for 8-14 Day Meal Plan

Meat & Poultry

Chicken thighs, boneless skinless – 400 g / 14 oz (Chicken Thighs with Dijon-Caper Sauce, Grilled Chicken Salad with Cauli Rice & Tahini)
Chicken breast – 200 g / 7 oz (Chicken and Cauliflower Rice Casserole with Broccoli)
Turkey sausage – 120 g / 4 oz (Egg White and Turkey Sausage Scramble)
Ground beef (lean) – 350 g / 12 oz (Vegetable and Ground Beef Stew with Zucchini, Eggplant Moussaka with Ground Beef and Parmesan)
Turkey breast, cubed or ground – 180 g / 6 oz (Turkey and Spinach Soup with Lemon)
Eggs – 16 large (Crustless Veggie Quiche with Bell Peppers and Onions, Mushroom and Asparagus Egg Bake, Hard-Boiled Eggs with Olive Tapenade, Buckwheat Pancakes with Cinnamon and Walnuts, Blueberry Almond Mug Cake)
Egg whites – 5 large (Egg White and Turkey Sausage Scramble)

Fish & Seafood

Salmon fillet – 180 g / 6 oz (Salmon Fillet with Pomegranate Glaze and Herbs)
Halibut fillet (or cod) – 180 g / 6 oz (Herb-Crusted Halibut with Cauliflower Mash)

Vegetables

Cauliflower – 2 medium heads (about 1.4 kg / 50 oz total) (Chicken and Cauliflower Rice Casserole with Broccoli, Creamy Cauliflower and Leek Soup with Roasted Garlic, Cauliflower Mash, Grilled Chicken Salad with Cauli Rice & Tahini)
Broccoli – 1 small head (about 300 g / 10 oz) (Chicken and Cauliflower Rice Casserole with Broccoli)
Bell peppers (red/yellow/green) – 4 large (Crustless Veggie Quiche with Bell Peppers and Onions, Vegetable and Ground Beef Stew with Zucchini)
Zucchini – 4 medium (Vegetable and Ground Beef Stew with Zucchini, Eggplant Moussaka with Ground Beef and Parmesan)
Eggplant – 3 large (Grilled Eggplant Salad with Yogurt-Tahini Dressing, Roasted Eggplant Salad with Tahini and Pomegranate, Eggplant Moussaka with Ground Beef and Parmesan)
Brussels sprouts – 250 g / 9 oz (Freekeh Bowl with Roasted Brussels Sprouts and Tahini Drizzle)
Leek – 2 medium (Creamy Cauliflower and Leek Soup with Roasted Garlic)
Asparagus – 1 large bunch (about 300 g / 10 oz) (Herb-Crusted Halibut with Cauliflower Mash, Beef

Wellington with Almond Flour Crust and Roasted Asparagus)
Onion – 3 medium (Crustless Veggie Quiche with Bell Peppers and Onions, Vegetable and Ground Beef Stew with Zucchini, Pumpkin and Cinnamon Smoothie)
Garlic – 2 bulbs (Creamy Cauliflower and Leek Soup with Roasted Garlic, Roasted Eggplant Salad with Tahini and Pomegranate, Grilled Chicken Salad with Cauli Rice & Tahini)
Fresh basil – 1 small bunch (Tomato and Red Lentil Soup with Fresh Basil)
Fresh parsley – 1 small bunch (Eggplant Moussaka with Ground Beef and Parmesan, Herb-Crusted Halibut with Cauliflower Mash)
Fresh mint – 1 small bunch (Grilled Eggplant Salad with Yogurt-Tahini Dressing)
Tomatoes – 7 medium (Tomato and Red Lentil Soup with Fresh Basil, Grilled Eggplant Salad, Grilled Chicken Salad)
Mixed salad greens – 1 small bag (100 g / 3.5 oz) (Grilled Chicken Salad with Cauli Rice & Tahini)
Pumpkin purée, unsweetened – 150 g / 2/3 cup (Pumpkin and Cinnamon Smoothie, Mini Chocolate Hazelnut Cakes, Keto Lemon Bars)

Fruits

Avocado – 3 large (Avocado and Chia Seed Smoothie, Grilled Chicken Salad with Cauli Rice & Tahini)
Apple – 2 medium (Low-Sugar Apple Spice Cake with Almond Flour)
Blueberries – 120 g / 1 cup (Berry Almond Quinoa Bowl, Blueberry Almond Mug Cake)
Pomegranate – 2 medium or 1 cup seeds (Salmon Fillet with Pomegranate Glaze and Herbs, Roasted Eggplant Salad with Tahini and Pomegranate)
Lemon – 4 medium (Turkey and Spinach Soup with Lemon, Herb-Crusted Halibut with Cauliflower Mash, Grilled Eggplant Salad, Grilled Chicken Salad)
Orange – 2 medium (Orange Almond Biscotti)

Grains & Bread

Quinoa, dry – 80 g / 1/2 cup (Berry Almond Quinoa Bowl)
Freekeh, dry – 80 g / 1/2 cup (Freekeh Bowl with Roasted Brussels Sprouts and Tahini Drizzle)
Buckwheat flour – 70 g / 1/2 cup (Buckwheat Pancakes with Cinnamon and Walnuts)
Almond flour – 300 g / 3 cups (Low-Sugar Apple Spice Cake with Almond Flour, Almond Flour Snickerdoodle Cookies, Mini Chocolate Hazelnut Cakes, Beef Wellington, Keto Lemon Bars, Orange Almond Biscotti)
Hazelnut flour (or finely ground hazelnuts) – 50 g / 1/2 cup (Mini Chocolate Hazelnut Cakes)
Whole wheat bread or baguette – 1 small loaf (Serve with soups/quiches if desired)

Dairy & Eggs

Greek yogurt, plain – 120 g / 1/2 cup (Grilled Eggplant Salad with Yogurt-Tahini Dressing)
Feta cheese – 100 g / 3.5 oz (Grilled Eggplant Salad with Yogurt-Tahini Dressing)
Parmesan cheese – 60 g / 2 oz (Eggplant Moussaka with Ground Beef and Parmesan)
Butter, unsalted – 90 g / 6 tbsp (Baking: Biscotti, Cakes, Beef Wellington crust)
Milk, unsweetened (dairy or plant-based) – 500 ml / 2 cups (Smoothies, Mug Cakes, Pancakes)

Nuts, Seeds & Nut Butter

Almonds, sliced or whole – 60 g / 1/2 cup (Berry Almond Quinoa Bowl, Blueberry Almond Mug Cake, Orange Almond Biscotti)
Hazelnuts, chopped – 40 g / 1/3 cup (Mini Chocolate Hazelnut Cakes)
Walnuts, chopped – 40 g / 1/3 cup (Buckwheat Pancakes with Cinnamon and Walnuts)
Chia seeds – 6 tbsp / 60 g (Avocado and Chia Seed Smoothie, Berry Almond Quinoa Bowl)
Tahini – 6 tbsp / 90 g (Freekeh Bowl, Roasted Eggplant Salad, Grilled Chicken Salad, Yogurt-Tahini Dressing)
Nut butter (almond or hazelnut) – 2 tbsp / 30 g (Smoothies, Mug Cakes)

Pantry Staples

Extra virgin olive oil – 120 ml / 1/2 cup (General, Roasting, Salads, Drizzles, Beef Wellington)

Grocery Shopping List for 15-21 Day Meal Plan

Meat & Poultry

Chicken breast – 350 g / 12 oz (Spinach & Feta Stuffed Chicken, Green Vegetable Stew with Chicken and Dill, Chicken and Lentil Stew)
Pork tenderloin – 200 g / 7 oz (Stuffed Pork Tenderloin with Spinach, Walnuts, and Goat Cheese)
Steak (sirloin or strip) – 180 g / 6 oz (Grilled Steak with Roasted Vegetables and Quinoa)
Duck breast – 180 g / 6 oz (Seared Duck Breast with Red Cabbage and Caraway)

Fish & Seafood

Octopus, cleaned – 200 g / 7 oz (Grilled Octopus with Arugula and Olive Oil)
Flounder fillets – 180 g / 6 oz (Baked Flounder with Broccoli and Cauliflower)
Smoked salmon – 100 g / 3.5 oz (Buckwheat Bowl with Smoked Salmon and Avocado)
Canned tuna in water – 1 can (120 g / 4 oz drained) (Tuna-Stuffed Avocados with Olive Oil and Lemon)

Vegetables

Eggplant – 3 medium (Eggplant Chickpea Stew with Tahini, Roasted Veggie Bowls, Roasted Vegetables for Steak)
Zucchini – 5 medium (Avocado & Egg Mash on Zucchini Rounds, Zucchini and Feta Omelet, Roasted Veggie Bowls)
Broccoli – 2 small heads (600 g / 21 oz total) (Creamy Broccoli and Cauliflower Soup with Almonds, Baked Flounder, Buckwheat and Roasted Broccoli Bowl)
Cauliflower – 2 small heads (700 g / 25 oz total) (Creamy Broccoli and Cauliflower Soup with Almonds, Baked Flounder, Cauliflower Steaks, Garlic and Herb Quinoa)
Spinach – 300 g / 10 oz (Spinach & Feta Stuffed Chicken, Spinach and Mushroom Egg Muffins, Almond Flour Crepes, Tofu Scramble, Omelets, Stuffed Pork Tenderloin)
Red cabbage – 1/2 head (350 g / 12 oz) (Seared Duck Breast with Red Cabbage and Caraway)
Mushrooms (cremini or button) – 250 g / 9 oz (Spinach and Mushroom Egg Muffins, Tofu Scramble)
Sweet mini peppers – 8–10 pieces (250 g / 9 oz) (Ricotta-Stuffed Sweet Mini Peppers)
Bell peppers (any color) – 4 medium (Tofu Scramble, Roasted Veggie Bowls, Omelets)
Onion – 2 medium (Lentil and Vegetable Skillet, Roasted Vegetables)
Avocado – 5 large (Avocado & Egg Mash on Zucchini Rounds, Buckwheat Bowl with Smoked Salmon and Avocado, Tuna-Stuffed Avocados)
Garlic – 2 bulbs (Eggplant Chickpea Stew, Cauliflower

Tomato paste – 2 tbsp / 30 g (Eggplant Moussaka, Stews)
Red lentils, dry – 80 g / 1/2 cup (Tomato and Red Lentil Soup with Fresh Basil)
Capers – 2 tbsp / 20 g (Chicken Thighs with Dijon-Caper Sauce)
Dijon mustard – 2 tbsp / 30 g (Chicken Thighs with Dijon-Caper Sauce)
Tapenade (olive spread) – 80 g / 3 oz (Hard-Boiled Eggs with Olive Tapenade)
Pomegranate molasses – 2 tbsp / 30 ml (Salmon Fillet with Pomegranate Glaze and Herbs, Roasted Eggplant Salad)
Cocoa powder – 2 tbsp / 20 g (Mini Chocolate Hazelnut Cakes)
Coconut flour – 30 g / 1/4 cup (Keto Lemon Bars)
Baking powder – 2 tsp (Mug Cakes, Pancakes, Baking)
Baking soda – 1 tsp (Biscotti, Cakes)
Vanilla extract – 2 tsp (Baking, Mug Cakes, Pancakes, Smoothies)
Ground cinnamon – 3 tsp (Apple Spice Cake, Pancakes, Pumpkin Smoothie, Snickerdoodle Cookies)
Ground nutmeg – 1 tsp (Apple Spice Cake, Pancakes)
Sweetener, erythritol or coconut sugar – 80 g / 1/3 cup (Low-Sugar Desserts, Cakes)
Dark chocolate chips – 60 g / 1/2 cup (Mini Chocolate Hazelnut Cakes, Blueberry Almond Mug Cake)
Salt and black pepper – to taste (General use)

Steaks, Roasted Veggie Bowls, Soups)
Arugula – 60 g / 2 oz (Grilled Octopus with Arugula and Olive Oil)
Dill, fresh – 1 small bunch (Green Vegetable Stew with Chicken and Dill)
Fresh herbs (parsley, thyme, chives) – 1 small bunch each (Herb Quinoa, Omelets, Lentil Skillet, Ricotta Cups)
Lemon – 5 medium (Mini Lemon Ricotta Cups, Tuna-Stuffed Avocados, Herb Quinoa, Grilled Octopus)

Fruits

Lemon (already included above)
Pecans – 40 g / 1/3 cup (Keto Pumpkin Pancakes)
Apple – 1 medium (Serve with breakfast or snacking, optional)

Grains & Bread

Quinoa, dry – 120 g / 2/3 cup (Grilled Steak with Roasted Vegetables and Quinoa, Cauliflower Steaks with Garlic and Herb Quinoa)
Buckwheat, dry or flour – 100 g / 2/3 cup (Buckwheat and Roasted Broccoli Bowl, Buckwheat Bowl with Smoked Salmon and Avocado)
Almond flour – 200 g / 2 cups (Almond Flour Crepes, Keto Chocolate Lava Cake, Mini Lemon Ricotta Cups)
Rolled oats – 40 g / 1/2 cup (Energy Balls, Ricotta Cups)

Dairy & Eggs

Eggs – 16 large (Cottage Cheese Omelet with Herbs, Spinach and Mushroom Egg Muffins, Keto Pumpkin Pancakes, Zucchini and Feta Omelet, Almond Flour Crepes, Avocado & Egg Mash)
Egg whites – 4 large (Tofu Scramble)
Cottage cheese – 250 g / 1 cup (Cottage Cheese Omelet, Cottage Cheese with Walnuts and Cinnamon)
Ricotta cheese – 200 g / 7 oz (Ricotta-Stuffed Sweet Mini Peppers, Almond Flour Crepes, Mini Lemon Ricotta Cups)
Goat cheese – 80 g / 3 oz (Stuffed Pork Tenderloin)
Feta cheese – 120 g / 4 oz (Spinach & Feta Stuffed Chicken, Zucchini and Feta Omelet)
Parmesan cheese – 50 g / 2 oz (Eggplant Chickpea Stew, Pasta garnish)
Greek yogurt, plain – 120 g / 1/2 cup (Ricotta cups, optional dressing)

Nuts, Seeds & Nut Butter

Almonds, whole or sliced – 50 g / 1/3 cup (Creamy Broccoli and Cauliflower Soup with Almonds)
Walnuts, chopped – 40 g / 1/3 cup (Cottage Cheese with Walnuts and Cinnamon, Stuffed Pork Tenderloin)
Sunflower seeds, hulled – 3 tbsp / 30 g (Buckwheat and Roasted Broccoli Bowl)
Tahini – 6 tbsp / 90 g (Eggplant Chickpea Stew, Quinoa and Roasted Veggie Bowl, Ricotta Cups, Avocado Mash)
Dark chocolate (70% or higher) – 100 g / 3.5 oz (Keto Chocolate Lava Cake, Mini Lemon Ricotta Cups)
Chia seeds – 2 tbsp / 20 g (Ricotta Cups, Avocado Mash)

Pantry Staples

Olive oil, extra virgin – 120 ml / 1/2 cup (General, Salads, Roasting, Sautéing)
Coconut oil – 3 tbsp / 45 ml (Energy Balls, Ricotta Cups, Pancakes, Lava Cake)
Pumpkin purée, unsweetened – 100 g / 1/2 cup (Keto Pumpkin Pancakes)
Chickpeas, cooked or canned – 200 g / 7 oz (Eggplant Chickpea Stew)
Lentils, dry (brown or green) – 100 g / 2/3 cup (Lentil and Vegetable Skillet, Chicken and Lentil Stew)
Red wine vinegar – 2 tbsp / 30 ml (Salads, Veggie Bowls)
Caraway seeds – 1 tsp (Seared Duck Breast with Red Cabbage)
Ground cinnamon – 2 tsp (Cottage Cheese with Walnuts and Cinnamon, Pumpkin Pancakes)
Baking powder – 1 tsp (Pumpkin Pancakes, Almond Flour Crepes)
Vanilla extract – 2 tsp (Mini Lemon Ricotta Cups, Lava Cake, Pancakes)
Coconut flakes, unsweetened – 2 tbsp / 15 g (Energy Balls, Ricotta Cups)
Salt and black pepper – to taste (General use)

Grocery Shopping List for 22-28 Day Meal Plan

Meat & Poultry

Chicken breast – 500 g / 1.1 lb (Buckwheat Bowl with Grilled Chicken and Avocado, Chicken Salad with Avocado and Chia Seeds, Spinach and Feta Stuffed Chicken Breasts, Eggplant & Chicken Casserole with Herb Yogurt, Chicken and Quinoa Soup with Spinach and Herbs)

Turkey breast, cooked or deli – 200 g / 7 oz (Barley and Roasted Red Pepper Bowl with Turkey, Turkey and Avocado Lettuce Wraps)

Eggs – 14 large (Spinach and Feta Scramble with Sautéed Mushrooms, Spinach Egg Bites with Cottage Cheese, Cabbage Stir-Fry with Eggs and Carrots, Sautéed Zucchini and Bell Pepper Frittata, Savory Quinoa Breakfast Bowl)

Fish & Seafood

Calamari, cleaned – 180 g / 6 oz (Grilled Calamari with Lemon and Arugula Salad)

Vegetables

Spinach – 300 g / 10 oz (Spinach and Feta Scramble, Chicken and Quinoa Soup, Spinach Egg Bites, Spinach and Feta Stuffed Chicken Breasts, Salads, Bowls)

Broccoli – 2 small heads (600 g / 21 oz) (Broccoli and Chickpea Salad, Baked Tofu with Steamed Broccoli, Salads, Side)

Zucchini – 4 medium (Sautéed Zucchini and Bell Pepper Frittata, Bowls, Salads)

Red bell pepper – 3 large (Sautéed Zucchini and Bell Pepper Frittata, Barley and Roasted Red Pepper Bowl, Roasted Veggies, Salads)

Yellow or orange bell pepper – 2 large (Frittata, Salads, Bowls)

Cucumber – 2 medium (Pumpkin Hummus with Cucumber, Salads)

Eggplant – 2 large (Eggplant & Chicken Casserole with Herb Yogurt)

Sweet potatoes – 2 medium (500 g / 1.1 lb) (Sweet Potato and Black Bean Salad with Lime-Cilantro Dressing)

Carrots – 3 medium (Cabbage Stir-Fry with Eggs and Carrots, Beef and Barley Soup with Root Vegetables)

Root vegetables (parsnip or turnip) – 2 small (Beef and Barley Soup with Root Vegetables)

Red onion – 2 medium (Salads, Roasted Veggies)

White onion – 1 medium (Beef and Barley Soup, Bowls)

Beets, cooked or raw – 2 medium (Roasted Beet and Goat Cheese Salad with Balsamic Glaze)

Cauliflower – 1 medium head (700 g / 25 oz) (Roasted Cauliflower and Chickpea Salad)

Cabbage (green or napa) – 1 small head (Cabbage Stir-Fry with Eggs and Carrots)

Lettuce leaves (romaine or butter) – 1 small head (Turkey and Avocado Lettuce Wraps)

Arugula – 60 g / 2 oz (Grilled Calamari with Lemon and Arugula Salad)

Fresh cilantro – 1 small bunch (Quinoa and Black Bean Bowl, Sweet Potato and Black Bean Salad)

Fresh parsley – 1 small bunch (Chicken and Quinoa Soup, Casserole, Bowls)

Fresh dill – 1 small bunch (Eggplant & Chicken Casserole with Herb Yogurt, Salad toppers)

Lemon – 5 medium (Grilled Calamari, Dressings, Salads, Yogurt Sauce, Bowls)

Lime – 2 medium (Quinoa and Black Bean Bowl, Sweet Potato Salad)

Garlic – 2 bulbs (Yogurt Dressings, Tahini Sauces, Roasting, Casseroles)

Fruits

Banana – 2 medium (Banana Nut Oat Bars with Almond Butter)

Strawberries – 180 g / 1.5 cups (Strawberry Almond Breakfast Smoothie)

Mixed berries (raspberries, blueberries, blackberries) – 250 g / 2 cups (Chia Seed Pudding with Coconut Milk and Raspberries, Keto-Friendly Berry Cheesecake Bars, Almond Coconut Ice Cream Bites)

Avocado – 4 large (Buckwheat Bowl with Grilled Chicken and Avocado, Chicken Salad with Avocado and Chia Seeds, Turkey and Avocado Lettuce Wraps)

Raspberries – 120 g / 1 cup (Chia Seed Pudding with Coconut Milk and Raspberries, Cheesecake Bars)

Grains & Bread

Quinoa, dry – 120 g / 2/3 cup (Quinoa and Black Bean Bowl, Chicken and Quinoa Soup, Savory Quinoa Breakfast Bowl, Pumpkin Spice Quinoa Porridge)
Barley, pearl – 80 g / 1/2 cup (Beef and Barley Soup with Root Vegetables, Barley and Roasted Red Pepper Bowl with Turkey)
Buckwheat, dry or flour – 80 g / 1/2 cup (Buckwheat Bowl with Grilled Chicken and Avocado)
Farro, dry – 70 g / 1/2 cup (Farro and Grilled Vegetables with a Yogurt-Tahini Dressing)
Oats, rolled – 80 g / 1 cup (Banana Nut Oat Bars with Almond Butter)

Dairy & Eggs

Greek yogurt, plain – 250 g / 1 cup (Quinoa and Black Bean Bowl, Farro and Grilled Vegetables, Dressings, Eggplant Casserole)
Yogurt, plain or coconut – 180 g / 3/4 cup (Broccoli and Chickpea Salad, Herb Yogurt Sauces)
Feta cheese – 120 g / 4 oz (Spinach and Feta Scramble, Spinach and Feta Stuffed Chicken Breasts)
Goat cheese – 60 g / 2 oz (Roasted Beet and Goat Cheese Salad)
Cottage cheese – 120 g / 1/2 cup (Spinach Egg Bites with Cottage Cheese)
Almond milk, unsweetened – 400 ml / 1.5 cups (Pumpkin Spice Quinoa Porridge, Smoothies, Chia Pudding)
Cream cheese, light or regular – 100 g / 3.5 oz (Keto-Friendly Berry Cheesecake Bars)

Nuts, Seeds & Nut Butter

Almonds, whole or sliced – 60 g / 1/2 cup (Strawberry Almond Breakfast Smoothie, Bars, Bowls)
Almond butter – 4 tbsp / 60 g (Banana Nut Oat Bars with Almond Butter)
Chia seeds – 8 tbsp / 80 g (Chia Seed Pudding with Coconut Milk and Raspberries, Chicken Salad with Avocado and Chia Seeds, Porridge, Bowls)
Sunflower seeds, hulled – 2 tbsp / 20 g (Salad toppers)
Pumpkin seeds – 2 tbsp / 20 g (Salad toppers, Bars)
Coconut flakes, unsweetened – 30 g / 1/3 cup (Almond Coconut Ice Cream Bites, Chia Pudding)
Pecans, chopped – 30 g / 1/4 cup (Oat Bars, Salad toppers)

Pantry Staples

Black beans, canned or cooked – 1 can (400 g / 14 oz) (Quinoa and Black Bean Bowl, Sweet Potato and Black Bean Salad)
Chickpeas, canned or cooked – 1 can (400 g / 14 oz) (Broccoli and Chickpea Salad, Roasted Cauliflower and Chickpea Salad)
Pumpkin purée, unsweetened – 120 g / 1/2 cup (Pumpkin Spice Quinoa Porridge, Pumpkin Hummus)
Tahini – 6 tbsp / 90 g (Yogurt-Tahini Dressings, Hummus, Bowls)
Coconut milk, canned – 1 can (400 ml / 14 oz) (Chia Seed Pudding, Ice Cream Bites)
Balsamic glaze or balsamic vinegar – 3 tbsp / 45 ml (Roasted Beet and Goat Cheese Salad)
Olive oil, extra virgin – 120 ml / 1/2 cup (General, Dressings, Sautéing, Roasting)
Dark chocolate (70% or higher) – 60 g / 1/2 bar (Berry Cheesecake Bars)
Honey or maple syrup – 2 tbsp / 30 ml (Cheesecake Bars, Yogurt Sauces)
Ground cinnamon – 2 tsp (Pumpkin Porridge, Bars, Breakfasts)
Vanilla extract – 2 tsp (Porridge, Smoothie, Cheesecake Bars, Bars)
Baking powder – 1 tsp (Bars, Cheesecake Bars)
Salt and black pepper – to taste (General use)

Grocery Shopping List for 29-35 Day Meal Plan

Meat & Poultry

Chicken breast – 350 g / 12 oz (Farro Bowl with Roasted Butternut Squash and Chicken, Grilled Chicken Salad with Avocado and Quinoa, Spaghetti Squash Casserole with Chicken and Alfredo Sauce)
Turkey tenderloin – 180 g / 6 oz (Grilled Turkey Tenderloin with Roasted Vegetables)
Ground turkey – 200 g / 7 oz (Butternut Squash and Zucchini

Lasagna with Turkey and Ricotta)

Fish & Seafood

Cod fillet – 180 g / 6 oz (Steamed Cod with Ginger-Garlic Cabbage)
Canned tuna in water – 1 can (120 g / 4 oz drained) (Stuffed Cherry Tomatoes with Avocado and Tuna)

Vegetables

Spinach – 350 g / 12 oz (Blueberry Spinach Smoothie with Flaxseeds, Spinach and Feta Crustless Quiche, Egg and Veggie Cups, Spinach and Strawberry Salad, Avocado and Tofu Breakfast Bowl, Spaghetti Squash Bowl, Hard-Boiled Eggs with Avocado and Spinach Salad, Bowls & Salads)
Kale – 120 g / 4 oz (Cucumber and Kale Smoothie)
Broccoli – 1 medium head (350 g / 12 oz) (Grilled Tofu with Sesame-Ginger Dressing and Broccoli, Broccoli and Avocado Salad with Lemon-Garlic Dressing)
Zucchini – 4 medium (Egg and Veggie Cups, Ratatouille, Butternut Squash and Zucchini Lasagna, Zucchini and Herb Soup, Zucchini Chips)
Butternut squash – 1 medium (600 g / 21 oz) (Farro Bowl, Lasagna)
Bell pepper (red, yellow, or orange) – 4 large (Egg and Veggie Cups, Ratatouille, Roasted Vegetables, Salads)
Cherry tomatoes – 200 g / 1.5 cups (Stuffed Cherry Tomatoes with Avocado and Tuna, Spinach Salad, Roasted Veg)
Tomatoes – 3 medium (Chard and Ricotta Bake, Salads, Ratatouille)
Cucumber – 3 medium (Avocado and Cucumber Salad, Salads, Smoothies)
Onion – 2 medium (Egg and Veggie Cups, Ratatouille, Roasted Veg)
Garlic – 2 bulbs (Dressing, Lasagna, Sautéing, Soup, Steamed Cod)
Green chard – 1 small bunch (200 g / 7 oz) (Chard and Ricotta Bake)
Lettuce or mixed greens – 100 g / 3.5 oz (Tofu Salad with Greens and Lemon-Oil Dressing)
Kale (listed above)
Avocado – 6 large (Avocado and Tofu Breakfast Bowl, Chicken & Avocado Pita Wedges, Broccoli and Avocado Salad, Salads, Bowls, Stuffed Tomatoes, Chicken Salad)
Spaghetti squash – 1 medium (600 g / 21 oz) (Spaghetti Squash Bowl with Roasted Chickpeas and Spinach, Spaghetti Squash Casserole with Chicken and Alfredo Sauce)
Lemon – 5 medium (Lemon-Garlic Dressing, Salads, Poached Egg, Dressings, Steamed Cod)
Lime – 2 medium (Avocado and Cucumber Salad with Lime-Cilantro Dressing)
Fresh cilantro – 1 small bunch (Avocado and Cucumber Salad)
Fresh parsley – 1 small bunch (Ratatouille, Zucchini and Herb Soup, General garnish)
Fresh ginger – 1 small knob (Sesame-Ginger Dressing, Steamed Cod)

Fruits

Blueberries – 120 g / 1 cup (Blueberry Spinach Smoothie with Flaxseeds)
Strawberries – 120 g / 1 cup (Spinach and Strawberry Salad)
Peaches – 2 medium (Cottage Cheese with Fresh Peaches and a Drizzle of Honey)
Lemon, lime (listed above)

Grains & Bread

Farro, dry – 70 g / 1/2 cup (Farro Bowl with Roasted Butternut Squash and Chicken)
Quinoa, dry – 80 g / 1/2 cup (Grilled Chicken Salad with Avocado and Quinoa)
Almond flour – 150 g / 1.5 cups (Spinach and Feta Crustless Quiche, No-Bake Coconut Almond Bars, Bites)
Pita bread, whole grain – 2 small rounds (Chicken & Avocado Pita Wedges)

Dairy & Eggs

Eggs – 14 large (Egg and Veggie Cups, Zucchini and Herb Soup with Poached Egg, Quiche, Breakfast Bowls, Lasagna, Salad, Hard-Boiled Eggs)
Ricotta cheese – 200 g / 7 oz (Chard and Ricotta Bake, Butternut Squash and Zucchini Lasagna, Spinach and Feta Crustless Quiche)

Feta cheese – 100 g / 3.5 oz (Spinach and Feta Crustless Quiche, Salads, Lasagna)
Cottage cheese – 120 g / 1/2 cup (Cottage Cheese with Fresh Peaches and a Drizzle of Honey)
Parmesan cheese – 60 g / 2 oz (Zucchini Chips with Parmesan Dust, Lasagna)
Greek yogurt, plain – 150 g / 2/3 cup (Salad dressings, Bowls, Alfredo Sauce)

Nuts, Seeds & Nut Butter

Almonds, whole or sliced – 40 g / 1/3 cup (No-Bake Coconut Almond Bars, Smoothies, Salads)
Flaxseeds, ground – 4 tbsp / 40 g (Blueberry Spinach Smoothie with Flaxseeds, Bowls)
Chia seeds – 2 tbsp / 20 g (Salad toppers, Bowls)
Coconut flakes, unsweetened – 40 g / 1/3 cup (Cacao Coconut Bites with Allulose, No-Bake Coconut Almond Bars)
Poppy seeds – 1 tbsp / 10 g (Spinach and Strawberry Salad with Poppy Seed Dressing)
Sesame seeds – 2 tbsp / 20 g (Grilled Tofu with Sesame-Ginger Dressing)

Pantry Staples

Chickpeas, cooked or canned – 1 can (400 g / 14 oz) (Spaghetti Squash Bowl with Roasted Chickpeas and Spinach)
Allulose or preferred sweetener – 2 tbsp / 20 g (Cacao Coconut Bites with Allulose)
Olive oil, extra virgin – 120 ml / 1/2 cup (Dressings, Roasting, Sautéing)
Honey – 2 tbsp / 30 ml (Cottage Cheese with Fresh Peaches, Dressings)
Almond butter – 2 tbsp / 30 g (Bars, Bowls)
Tahini – 4 tbsp / 60 g (Salads, Dressings, Bowls)
Coconut oil – 2 tbsp / 30 ml (Bites, Bars)
Sesame oil – 1 tbsp / 15 ml (Sesame-Ginger Dressing)
Balsamic vinegar – 2 tbsp / 30 ml (Salad Dressings)
Salt and black pepper – to taste (General use)

Grocery Shopping List for 36-42 Day Meal Plan

Meat & Poultry

Chicken drumsticks – 400 g / 14 oz (Baked Chicken Drumsticks with Veggie Sauté)
Chicken breast – 180 g / 6 oz (Walnut-Crusted Chicken with Garlic Green Beans)
Ground beef – 250 g / 9 oz (Mushroom and Ground Beef Casserole with Cauliflower, Root Vegetable and Beef Stew)
Flank steak – 180 g / 6 oz (Grilled Flank Steak with Quinoa and Roasted Brussels Sprouts)
Turkey breast, cooked or deli – 180 g / 6 oz (Grilled Turkey and Mixed Greens Salad with Mustard Vinaigrette)
Ground turkey – 200 g / 7 oz (Turkey Meatloaf Roll with Mushrooms)

Fish & Seafood

(No main fish/seafood this week; skip unless desired as extra.)

Vegetables

Spinach – 250 g / 9 oz (Egg Muffins, Kale and Spinach Hummus, Eggplant Rollatini, Orange and Spinach Salad, Bowls)
Kale – 150 g / 5 oz (Warm Kale and Quinoa Breakfast Bowl, Kale and Spinach Hummus)
Zucchini – 6 medium (Zucchini and Egg Casserole, Zucchini and Mushroom Lasagna, Zucchini and Egg Protein Bowl, Bowls, Casseroles)
Bell peppers (red, yellow, green) – 5 large (Egg Muffins, Stuffed Bell Peppers, Bowls, Sauté)
Mushrooms (button or cremini) – 350 g / 12 oz (Tofu and Mushroom Crustless Pie, Turkey Meatloaf Roll, Zucchini and Mushroom Lasagna, Casseroles)
Eggplant – 2 large (Eggplant Rollatini with Ricotta and Spinach)
Cauliflower – 2 small heads (700 g / 25 oz total) (Cauliflower Gratin, Mushroom and Ground Beef Casserole, Stuffed Peppers)
Broccoli – 2 small heads (600 g / 21 oz total) (Mini Broccoli and Cheese Casserole)
Brussels sprouts – 250 g / 9 oz (Grilled Flank Steak with Quinoa and Roasted Brussels Sprouts)
Asparagus – 1 bunch (200 g / 7 oz) (Asparagus and Goat Cheese Omelette)

Green beans – 200 g / 7 oz (Walnut-Crusted Chicken with Garlic Green Beans)
Root vegetables (carrot, parsnip, turnip) – 4 medium (Root Vegetable and Beef Stew, Veggie Sauté)
Onion – 3 medium (Egg Muffins, Sauté, Casseroles, Bowls)
Garlic – 2 bulbs (General, Hummus, Bowls, Sauté, Pesto, Stews)
Fresh herbs (basil, parsley, dill, oregano) – 1 bunch each (Omelettes, Pesto, Lasagna, Bowls, Garnishes)
Radish – 5–6 medium (Radish Slices with Herbed Cream Cheese)
Lime – 2 medium (Chicken and Chickpea Salad with Avocado and Lime)
Lemon – 4 medium (Salad, Bowls, Hummus, Parfait)
Mixed greens or arugula – 100 g / 3.5 oz (Grilled Turkey Salad, Salads)
Avocado – 3 large (Chicken and Chickpea Salad, Stuffed Peppers, Bowls)
Cherry tomatoes – 150 g / 1 cup (Stuffed Cherry Tomatoes, Salads, Bowls)

Fruits

Strawberries – 120 g / 1 cup (Strawberry and Coconut Cream Chia Parfait)
Banana – 1 medium (Banana Almond Mug Muffin)
Orange – 1 medium (Orange and Spinach Salad with Almonds)
Berries (mixed, for parfait/pudding) – 150 g / 1 cup (Coconut Chia Pudding with Berries, Parfait)

Grains & Bread

Quinoa, dry – 100 g / 2/3 cup (Warm Kale and Quinoa Breakfast Bowl, Flank Steak Bowl, Grilled Chicken Salad, Bowls)
Barley, pearl – 50 g / 1/3 cup (Bowls, optional swap in sides)
Almond flour – 200 g / 2 cups (Lemon Poppy Seed Muffins, Almond Flour Crackers, Mug Muffin)
Whole grain pita bread – 2 rounds (Low-Carb Pita with Basil Pesto and Feta)

Dairy & Eggs

Eggs – 16 large (Egg Muffins, Protein Bowls, Omelettes, Casseroles, Lasagna, Greek Bowl)
Gruyère cheese – 80 g / 3 oz (Cauliflower Gratin)
Cheddar or mozzarella cheese – 120 g / 4 oz (Mini Broccoli and Cheese Casserole, Lasagna)
Feta cheese – 120 g / 4 oz (Zucchini and Egg Casserole, Low-Carb Pita, Greek Bowl)
Ricotta cheese – 150 g / 5 oz (Eggplant Rollatini, Lasagna)
Cream cheese – 80 g / 3 oz (Radish Slices with Herbed Cream Cheese)
Goat cheese – 60 g / 2 oz (Asparagus and Goat Cheese Omelette)
Greek yogurt, plain – 120 g / 1/2 cup (Bowls, Salads, Parfait)
Milk or almond milk, unsweetened – 400 ml / 1.5 cups (Gratin, Muffins, Puddings)

Nuts, Seeds & Nut Butter

Almonds, sliced or whole – 40 g / 1/3 cup (Orange and Spinach Salad, Muffin, Crackers)
Chia seeds – 6 tbsp / 60 g (Coconut Chia Pudding, Strawberry Parfait)
Poppy seeds – 1 tbsp / 10 g (Lemon Poppy Seed Muffins)
Walnuts, chopped – 40 g / 1/3 cup (Walnut-Crusted Chicken, Bowls, Salads)

Pantry Staples

Black beans, canned or cooked – 1 can (400 g / 14 oz) (Stuffed Bell Peppers)
Chickpeas, cooked or canned – 1 can (400 g / 14 oz) (Chicken and Chickpea Salad, Hummus)
Coconut milk, canned – 1 can (400 ml / 14 oz) (Coconut Chia Pudding, Parfait)
Coconut cream – 50 ml / 3 tbsp (Strawberry and Coconut Cream Chia Parfait)
Almond butter – 2 tbsp / 30 g (Banana Almond Mug Muffin, Bowls)
Tahini – 4 tbsp / 60 g (Hummus, Bowls)
Olives, black or green – 50 g / 1/4 cup (Savory Greek Bowl)
Olive oil, extra virgin – 120 ml / 1/2 cup (Dressings, Roasting, Sautéing)
Mustard, Dijon – 1 tbsp / 15 g (Mustard Vinaigrette)
Honey or allulose – 2 tbsp / 30 ml (Muffins, Bowls, Parfait)
Baking powder – 1.5 tsp (Muffins, Crackers, Mug Muffin)

Salt and black pepper – to taste (General use)
Basil pesto – 2 tbsp / 30 g (Low-Carb Pita with Basil Pesto and Feta)
Oregano, dried – 1 tsp (Casserole, Lasagna, Bowls)

Grocery Shopping List for 43-49 Day Meal Plan

Meat & Poultry

Chicken breast – 400 g / 14 oz (Sliced Chicken Breast with Guacamole and Veggies, Brussels Sprouts and Chicken Casserole with Almond Crust, Herb-Roasted Whole Chicken with Garlic and Lemon)
Whole chicken – 1 small (about 1.2 kg / 2.6 lb) (Herb-Roasted Whole Chicken with Garlic and Lemon)
Ground beef – 200 g / 7 oz (French-Style Baked Meat, Beef Roll with Spinach, Feta & Eggplant)
Sirloin steak – 180 g / 6 oz (Grilled Sirloin with Cauli Rice & Asparagus)
Pork loin – 180 g / 6 oz (Pork Loin with Apple & Sage)
Turkey breast or thigh – 180 g / 6 oz (Turkey and Cabbage Stir-Fry)

Fish & Seafood

Trout fillet – 180 g / 6 oz (Baked Trout with Roasted Fennel and Lemon)
Salmon fillet or canned – 180 g / 6 oz (Roasted Salmon Cakes with Yogurt Dill Sauce)
Canned tuna in water – 1 can (120 g / 4 oz drained) (Avocado Tuna Boats)

Vegetables

Spinach – 250 g / 9 oz (Sweet Potato and Spinach Hash with Egg, Beef Roll with Spinach, Feta & Eggplant, Cauliflower and Egg Power Bowl, Chickpea and Kale Stir-Fry with Garlic and Lemon, Spinach and Ricotta Stuffed Mushrooms, Brussels Sprouts and Chicken Casserole with Almond Crust, Power Bowls, Salads)
Kale – 120 g / 4 oz (Chickpea and Kale Stir-Fry with Garlic and Lemon)
Cabbage (green or napa) – 1 small head (Turkey and Cabbage Stir-Fry, Cabbage and Tofu Bake with Almond Crumble)
Eggplant – 5 medium (Grilled Eggplant Steaks with Herbed Yogurt Sauce, Eggplant Breakfast Pizza with Scrambled Eggs and Parmesan, Beef Roll with Spinach, Feta & Eggplant, Eggplant and Goat Cheese Stack)
Zucchini – 6 medium (Beetroot Hummus with Carrot and Zucchini Ribbons, Olive and Sun-Dried Tomato Hummus with Zucchini, Nutty Green Smoothie with Zucchini and Almonds, Crustless Zucchini Pie with Goat Cheese and Dill, Power Bowls, Ribbons, Sides)
Bell peppers (red, yellow, or orange) – 4 large (Stuffed Bell Peppers with Quinoa, Chickpeas, and Herbs)
Sweet potato – 2 medium (500 g / 1.1 lb) (Sweet Potato and Spinach Hash with Egg)
Carrots – 2 medium (Beetroot Hummus with Carrot and Zucchini Ribbons, Cauliflower Tabbouleh, Power Bowls)
Cauliflower – 2 small heads (700 g / 25 oz total) (Cauliflower Tabbouleh with Cucumber, Tomato, and Mint, Cauliflower and Egg Power Bowl, Grilled Sirloin with Cauli Rice & Asparagus, Stuffed Bell Peppers, Casserole)
Broccoli – 1 small head (300 g / 10 oz) (Power Bowls, Sides, Casseroles)
Brussels sprouts – 250 g / 9 oz (Brussels Sprouts and Chicken Casserole with Almond Crust)
Fennel – 1 bulb (Baked Trout with Roasted Fennel and Lemon)
Tomatoes – 3 medium (Cauliflower Tabbouleh, Power Bowls, Salads)
Cherry tomatoes – 150 g / 1 cup (Cauliflower Tabbouleh, Salads, Sides)
Cucumber – 2 medium (Cauliflower Tabbouleh, Salads, Sides)
Lettuce or mixed greens – 100 g / 3.5 oz (Salads, Sides)
Avocado – 4 large (Avocado Tuna Boats, Sliced Chicken Breast with Guacamole and Veggies, Power Bowls, Guacamole)
Beetroot, cooked or raw – 2 small (Beetroot Hummus with Carrot and Zucchini Ribbons)
Fresh parsley – 1 small bunch (Stuffed Bell Peppers, Power Bowls, Stews, Гарниш)

Fresh mint – 1 small bunch (Cauliflower Tabbouleh)
Fresh dill – 1 small bunch (Yogurt Dill Sauce, Power Bowls)
Fresh sage – 1 small bunch (Pork Loin with Apple & Sage)
Lemon – 5 medium (Herb-Roasted Whole Chicken with Garlic and Lemon, Grilled Eggplant Steaks with Herbed Yogurt Sauce, Yogurt Dill Sauce, Fish, Power Bowls, Salads)
Lime – 2 medium (Guacamole, Salads, Dressings)
Garlic – 2 bulbs (General, Stews, Bowls, Roasts, Dressings, Sauces)
Onion – 3 medium (French-Style Baked Meat, Cabbage and Tofu Bake, Pilaf, Stews, Sides, Casseroles, Hash)

Fruits

Apple – 2 medium (Pork Loin with Apple & Sage, Apple Cinnamon Overnight Oats with Flaxseeds)
Strawberries – 120 g / 1 cup (Low-Carb Strawberry Shortcake Cups)
Berries (mixed, for cups) – 120 g / 1 cup (Low-Carb Strawberry Shortcake Cups)

Grains & Bread

Quinoa, dry – 100 g / 2/3 cup (Stuffed Bell Peppers with Quinoa, Chickpeas, and Herbs, Power Bowls, Sides)
Brown rice, dry – 80 g / 1/2 cup (Pilaf with Brown Rice)
Oats, rolled – 80 g / 1 cup (Apple Cinnamon Overnight Oats with Flaxseeds)
Almond flour – 180 g / 1.5 cups (Low-Carb Strawberry Shortcake Cups, Almond Crumble for Cabbage and Tofu Bake)

Dairy & Eggs

Eggs – 14 large (Eggplant Breakfast Pizza with Scrambled Eggs and Parmesan, Cauliflower and Egg Power Bowl, Crustless Zucchini Pie with Goat Cheese and Dill, Spinach and Ricotta Stuffed Mushrooms, Beef Roll with Spinach, Feta & Eggplant, Brussels Sprouts and Chicken Casserole, Protein Bowls, Scrambled Eggs, Sides)
Ricotta cheese – 120 g / 4 oz (Spinach and Ricotta Stuffed Mushrooms, Butternut Squash and Zucchini Lasagna with Turkey and Ricotta, Crustless Zucchini Pie with Goat Cheese and Dill)
Goat cheese – 100 g / 3.5 oz (Crustless Zucchini Pie with Goat Cheese and Dill, Eggplant and Goat Cheese Stack)
Feta cheese – 80 g / 3 oz (Beef Roll with Spinach, Feta & Eggplant, Stuffed Bell Peppers with Quinoa, Chickpeas, and Herbs, Salads)
Parmesan cheese – 80 g / 3 oz (Eggplant Breakfast Pizza with Scrambled Eggs and Parmesan, Grilled Eggplant Steaks with Herbed Yogurt Sauce)
Yogurt, plain Greek or regular – 150 g / 2/3 cup (Herbed Yogurt Sauce, Yogurt Dill Sauce, Power Bowls, Parfaits, Dressings)
Gruyère cheese or mozzarella – 60 g / 2 oz (Cabbage and Tofu Bake with Almond Crumble, Casseroles)

Nuts, Seeds & Nut Butter

Almonds, whole or sliced – 40 g / 1/3 cup (Nutty Green Smoothie with Zucchini and Almonds, Low-Carb Strawberry Shortcake Cups)
Flaxseeds, ground – 4 tbsp / 40 g (Apple Cinnamon Overnight Oats with Flaxseeds, Bowls, Smoothies)
Sunflower seeds – 2 tbsp / 20 g (Salads, Power Bowls, Tabbouleh)

Pantry Staples

Chickpeas, cooked or canned – 2 cans (400 g / 14 oz each) (Chickpea and Kale Stir-Fry with Garlic and Lemon, Stuffed Bell Peppers with Quinoa, Chickpeas, and Herbs, Beetroot Hummus with Carrot and Zucchini Ribbons, Cauliflower Tabbouleh with Cucumber, Tomato, and Mint, Olive and Sun-Dried Tomato Hummus with Zucchini)
Black beans, cooked or canned – 1 can (400 g / 14 oz) (Stuffed Bell Peppers with Quinoa, Chickpeas, and Herbs, swaps)
Tahini – 4 tbsp / 60 g (Beetroot Hummus with Carrot and Zucchini Ribbons, Olive and Sun-Dried Tomato Hummus with Zucchini, Power Bowls, Dressings)

Coconut cream – 50 ml / 3 tbsp (Low-Carb Strawberry Shortcake Cups)
Honey or maple syrup – 2 tbsp / 30 ml (Apple Cinnamon Overnight Oats with Flaxseeds, Low-Carb Strawberry Shortcake Cups, Bowls)
Olive oil, extra virgin – 120 ml / 1/2 cup (Dressings, Roasting, Sautéing, Marinades)
Sun-dried tomatoes in oil – 40 g / 1/4 cup (Olive and Sun-Dried Tomato Hummus with Zucchini, Salads, Bowls)
Poppy seeds – 1 tbsp / 10 g (Apple Cinnamon Overnight Oats with Flaxseeds, Tabbouleh)
Salt and black pepper – to taste (General use)

Grocery Shopping List for 50-56 Day Meal Plan

Meat & Poultry

Ground turkey – 600 g / 1.3 lb (Bulgur Wheat Bowl with Ground Turkey and Zucchini, Butternut Squash and Turkey Chili, Turkey and Black Bean Chili with Avocado, Baked Zucchini Turkey Fritters, Turkey and Veggie Breakfast Patties, Ground Turkey and Kale Casserole with Almond Crust, Millet and Carrot Bowl with Turkey Meatballs, Broccoli and Turkey Breakfast Bake with Cheddar)
Turkey breast, cooked or deli – 200 g / 7 oz (Turkey and Cucumber Roll-Ups with Mustard Dip)

Chicken breast – 200 g / 7 oz (Chicken and Chickpea Salad with Avocado and Lime)
Beef stew meat or ground beef – 300 g / 11 oz (Cabbage and Beef Tomato Stew, Shepherd's Pie with Cauliflower Mash)

Fish & Seafood

Scallops – 180 g / 6 oz (Lemon-Parsley Scallops with Sautéed Zucchini)
Mackerel, fresh or fillet – 180 g / 6 oz (Broiled Mackerel with Sautéed Spinach)
Smoked salmon – 120 g / 4 oz (Deviled Eggs with Smoked Salmon and Avocado Mousse, Smoked Salmon Rolls with Cucumber and Cream Cheese)
Canned tuna in water – 1 can (120 g / 4 oz drained) (Tuna Niçoise Salad with Hard-Boiled Eggs and Olive Oil)

Vegetables

Zucchini – 7 medium (Bulgur Wheat Bowl, Baked Zucchini Turkey Fritters, Lemon-Parsley Scallops, Low-Carb Zucchini Fritters, Power Bowls, Salads, Sauté)
Butternut squash – 1 medium (600 g / 21 oz) (Butternut Squash and Turkey Chili)
Acorn squash – 1 medium (Stuffed Acorn Squash with Wild Rice and Cranberries)
Cauliflower – 2 small heads (700 g / 25 oz total) (Millet and Roasted Cauliflower Bowl, Shepherd's Pie with Cauliflower Mash, Egg and Cauliflower Skillet, Casserole)

Cabbage (green or napa) – 1 small head (Cabbage and Beef Tomato Stew, Salads)
Kale – 120 g / 4 oz (Ground Turkey and Kale Casserole, Soft-Boiled Eggs with Sautéed Kale and Mushrooms, Bowls)
Spinach – 250 g / 9 oz (Broiled Mackerel with Sautéed Spinach, Egg and Cauliflower Skillet, Salads)
Baby spinach – 60 g / 2 oz (Egg and Cauliflower Skillet, Bowls, Sides)
Carrots – 3 medium (Millet and Carrot Bowl, Power Bowls, Stew, Salads)
Broccoli – 1 small head (300 g / 10 oz) (Broccoli and Turkey Breakfast Bake with Cheddar, Bowls)
Bell peppers (red/yellow/green) – 3 large (Cilantro Lime Hummus with Bell Pepper Strips, Power Bowls, Sides)
Onion – 3 medium (Chili, Stew, Casseroles, Fritters, Salads)
Mushrooms (button or cremini) – 200 g / 7 oz (Soft-Boiled Eggs with Sautéed Kale and Mushrooms, Sautéed, Bowls)
Cucumber – 3 medium (Turkey and Cucumber Roll-Ups, Smoked Salmon Rolls, Salads)
Avocado – 5 large (Chicken and Chickpea Salad, Turkey and Black Bean Chili, Deviled Eggs, Power Bowls, Salads)
Lemon – 5 medium (Lemon-Parsley Scallops, Vinaigrette, Salads, Hummus, Bowls)
Lime – 2 medium (Chicken and Chickpea Salad, Hummus, Salads)

Fresh parsley – 1 small bunch (Lemon-Parsley Scallops, Salads, Chili, Casseroles)
Fresh cilantro – 1 small bunch (Spinach and Quinoa Salad, Hummus, Salads)
Fresh dill – 1 small bunch (Salads, Dips, Power Bowls)
Garlic – 2 bulbs (General, Casseroles, Hummus, Chili, Dressings)

Fruits

Strawberries – 120 g / 1 cup (Strawberry Coconut Yogurt Bark, Warm Chia Almond Porridge with Berries)
Banana – 2 medium (Coconut Flour Banana Bread with Chia Seeds)
Berries (mixed, for bark and porridge) – 150 g / 1 cup (Strawberry Coconut Yogurt Bark, Warm Chia Almond Porridge with Berries)

Grains & Bread

Bulgur wheat, dry – 80 g / 1/2 cup (Bulgur Wheat Bowl with Ground Turkey and Zucchini)
Millet, dry – 80 g / 1/2 cup (Millet and Carrot Bowl with Turkey Meatballs, Millet and Roasted Cauliflower Bowl with Lemon Vinaigrette)
Wild rice, dry – 50 g / 1/3 cup (Stuffed Acorn Squash with Wild Rice and Cranberries)
Quinoa, dry – 80 g / 1/2 cup (Spinach and Quinoa Salad with Sunflower Seeds and Lemon Zest)
Coconut flour – 90 g / 3/4 cup (Coconut Flour Vanilla Cupcakes with Greek Yogurt Frosting, Coconut Flour Banana Bread with Chia Seeds)
Sunflower seeds – 2 tbsp / 20 g (Spinach and Quinoa Salad with Sunflower Seeds and Lemon Zest)

Dairy & Eggs

Eggs – 16 large (Soft-Boiled Eggs with Sautéed Kale and Mushrooms, Deviled Eggs with Smoked Salmon and Avocado Mousse, bakes, casseroles, fritters, patties, poached eggs, cupcakes, salad)
Greek yogurt, plain – 200 g / 7 oz (Coconut Flour Vanilla Cupcakes with Greek Yogurt Frosting, frosting, salads, bowls)
Cream cheese – 60 g / 2 oz (Smoked Salmon Rolls with Cucumber and Cream Cheese, Deviled Eggs with Smoked Salmon and Avocado Mousse)
Cheddar cheese – 80 g / 3 oz (Broccoli and Turkey Breakfast Bake with Cheddar)

Nuts, Seeds & Nut Butter

Almonds, whole or sliced – 40 g / 1/3 cup (Warm Chia Almond Porridge with Berries, bowls)
Chia seeds – 8 tbsp / 80 g (Coconut Flour Banana Bread with Chia Seeds, Warm Chia Almond Porridge with Berries, Strawberry Coconut Yogurt Bark)
Sunflower seeds – 2 tbsp / 20 g (Spinach and Quinoa Salad with Sunflower Seeds and Lemon Zest)

Pantry Staples

Black beans, canned or cooked – 1 can (400 g / 14 oz) (Turkey and Black Bean Chili with Avocado)
Chickpeas, canned or cooked – 2 cans (400 g / 14 oz each) (Chicken and Chickpea Salad with Avocado and Lime, millet bowls, salads, hummus)
Cranberries, dried – 30 g / 1/4 cup (Stuffed Acorn Squash with Wild Rice and Cranberries)
Coconut yogurt, unsweetened – 100 g / 1/2 cup (Strawberry Coconut Yogurt Bark)
Coconut oil – 2 tbsp / 30 ml (Strawberry Coconut Yogurt Bark, baking)
Olive oil, extra virgin – 120 ml / 1/2 cup (General, roasting, sautéing, dressings)
Honey or maple syrup – 2 tbsp / 30 ml (Coconut Flour Vanilla Cupcakes with Greek Yogurt Frosting, Coconut Flour Banana Bread with Chia Seeds, Warm Chia Almond Porridge with Berries)
Mustard, Dijon – 1 tbsp / 15 g (Turkey and Cucumber Roll-Ups with Mustard Dip, salads)
Salt and black pepper – to taste (General use)

Grocery Shopping List for 57-60 Day Meal Plan

Meat & Poultry

Chicken breast – 200 g / 7 oz (Barley Bowl with Roasted Fennel and Chicken)

Turkey bacon – 120 g / 4 oz (Egg and Spinach Breakfast Muffins with Turkey Bacon)
Sirloin steak – 180 g / 6 oz (Grilled Sirloin with Cauli Rice & Asparagus)
Beef stew meat – 250 g / 9 oz (Savory Beef and Mushroom Stew with Fresh Thyme)

Fish & Seafood

(No main fish/seafood this week; skip unless desired as extra.)

Vegetables

Spinach – 200 g / 7 oz (Egg and Spinach Breakfast Muffins with Turkey Bacon, Crustless Quiche with Spinach, Mushrooms, and Feta)
Broccoli – 1 small head (300 g / 10 oz) (Broccoli and Cheddar Scramble with Herbs)
Leek – 2 medium (Creamy Turnip and Leek Soup)
Turnip – 2 medium (Creamy Turnip and Leek Soup)
Zucchini – 4 medium (Crustless Zucchini Pie with Goat Cheese and Dill, Zucchini Rollatini with Ricotta and Walnut Filling)
Fennel – 1 bulb (Barley Bowl with Roasted Fennel and Chicken)
Cabbage (green or napa) – 1 small head (Tofu and Cabbage Stir-Fry with Ginger-Garlic Sauce)
Mushrooms (button or cremini) – 350 g / 12 oz (Savory Beef and Mushroom Stew with Fresh Thyme, Amaranth and Mushroom Bowl with Herb Yogurt Sauce, Crustless Quiche with Spinach, Mushrooms, and Feta)
Asparagus – 1 bunch (200 g / 7 oz) (Grilled Sirloin with Cauli Rice & Asparagus)
Onion – 2 medium (Stir-Fries, Quiches, Bowls, Stews)
Garlic – 2 bulbs (Tofu and Cabbage Stir-Fry with Ginger-Garlic Sauce, Bowls, Quiches, General)
Fresh dill – 1 small bunch (Crustless Zucchini Pie with Goat Cheese and Dill)
Fresh thyme – 1 small bunch (Savory Beef and Mushroom Stew with Fresh Thyme)
Herbs (parsley, chives, basil) – 1 small bunch each (Broccoli and Cheddar Scramble with Herbs, Amaranth and Mushroom Bowl)

Fruits

Raspberries – 120 g / 1 cup (Buckwheat Porridge with Almonds and Raspberries, Coconut Raspberry Thumbprint Cookies)
Lemon – 4 medium (Keto-Friendly Lemon Coconut Cake, Barley Bowl with Roasted Fennel and Chicken, Bowls, Dressings)
Pumpkin purée – 100 g / 1/2 cup (Sugar-Free Pumpkin Spice Cupcakes with Cream Cheese Frosting)

Grains & Bread

Buckwheat groats, dry – 70 g / 1/2 cup (Buckwheat Porridge with Almonds and Raspberries)
Barley, pearl – 70 g / 1/2 cup (Barley Bowl with Roasted Fennel and Chicken)
Amaranth, dry – 70 g / 1/2 cup (Amaranth and Mushroom Bowl with Herb Yogurt Sauce)

Dairy & Eggs

Eggs – 14 large (Egg and Spinach Breakfast Muffins with Turkey Bacon, Crustless Zucchini Pie with Goat Cheese and Dill, Crustless Quiche with Spinach, Mushrooms, and Feta, Scrambles, Muffins, Cupcakes)
Cheddar cheese – 80 g / 3 oz (Broccoli and Cheddar Scramble with Herbs)
Feta cheese – 80 g / 3 oz (Crustless Quiche with Spinach, Mushrooms, and Feta)
Ricotta cheese – 100 g / 3.5 oz (Zucchini Rollatini with Ricotta and Walnut Filling)
Goat cheese – 80 g / 3 oz (Crustless Zucchini Pie with Goat Cheese and Dill)
Cream cheese – 80 g / 3 oz (Sugar-Free Pumpkin Spice Cupcakes with Cream Cheese Frosting)
Greek yogurt, plain – 100 g / 1/2 cup (Amaranth and Mushroom Bowl with Herb Yogurt Sauce)

Nuts, Seeds & Nut Butter

Almonds, whole or sliced – 40 g / 1/3 cup (Buckwheat Porridge with Almonds and Raspberries, Coconut Raspberry Thumbprint Cookies)
Walnuts, chopped – 30 g / 1/4 cup (Zucchini Rollatini with Ricotta and Walnut Filling)
Pecans, chopped – 40 g / 1/3 cup (Keto Maple Pecan Scones)

Chia seeds – 2 tbsp / 20 g (Porridge, Bowls)
Coconut flakes, unsweetened – 40 g / 1/3 cup (Keto-Friendly Lemon Coconut Cake, Coconut Raspberry Thumbprint Cookies)

Pantry Staples

Coconut flour – 70 g / 2/3 cup (Keto-Friendly Lemon Coconut Cake, Sugar-Free Pumpkin Spice Cupcakes, Keto Maple Pecan Scones)
Maple syrup, sugar-free or regular – 2 tbsp / 30 ml (Keto Maple Pecan Scones)
Sugar substitute or sweetener – as needed (Keto-Friendly Lemon Coconut Cake, Sugar-Free Pumpkin Spice Cupcakes, Coconut Raspberry Thumbprint Cookies)
Olive oil, extra virgin – 120 ml / 1/2 cup (Roasting, sautéing, dressings, bowls)
Baking powder – 1.5 tsp (Scones, Cakes, Muffins)
Salt and black pepper – to taste (General use)
Vanilla extract – 2 tsp (Cakes, Cookies)

Personalized Health Journal

Managing diabetes isn't just about eating the right foods—it's about understanding how your body responds to daily choices, including diet, exercise, hydration, and rest. This **Personalized Diabetes Journal** is designed to empower you with insights into your health, allowing you to track key factors that influence blood sugar levels and overall well-being.

How to Use This Journal

By logging important health indicators daily or weekly, you can **spot trends, make informed adjustments, and improve diabetes management**. Regular tracking helps you refine your habits for **better blood sugar stability and long-term success**.

What to Track in Your Health Journal

📌 **Blood Sugar Readings**	📌 **Meals & Snacks**
• Record fasting, pre-meal, and post-meal glucose levels. • Identify patterns and adjust your meals, activity, or medication as needed.	• Keep a log of everything you eat and drink. • Note portion sizes, ingredients, and how your body reacts.
📌 **Physical Activity**	📌 **Hydration**
• Track workouts, walks, or any movement throughout the day. • Observe how exercise impacts your blood sugar and energy levels.	• Log your daily water intake. • Staying hydrated supports kidney function and helps regulate blood sugar.
📌 **Sleep Patterns**	📌 **Mood & Energy Levels**
• Track how many hours you sleep and the quality of rest. • Poor sleep can disrupt insulin sensitivity and lead to fatigue.	• Monitor how you feel emotionally and physically throughout the day. • Identify any links between mood changes, diet, stress, or activity.
📌 **Medications & Supplements**	
• Keep track of prescribed medications, insulin, and supplements. • Record any adjustments or side effects.	

Why Tracking Helps You Stay in Control

✔ **Recognize Blood Sugar Trends:** Find out which habits improve or disrupt glucose levels.
✔ **Optimize Meal Planning:** Learn which foods help keep your blood sugar stable.
✔ **Enhance Medical Appointments:** Provide clear health data for better treatment recommendations.
✔ **Stay Motivated:** Seeing progress in your health keeps you accountable and committed.

Set Your Weekly Health Goals

At the start of each week, write down simple, **achievable health goals** that align with your diabetes management plan. Examples include:

- Cutting back on refined carbs at dinner.
- Taking a 30-minute walk daily.
- Increasing daily water intake.
- Establishing a consistent bedtime routine.

By **consistently tracking and setting goals**, you'll develop a deeper understanding of what works best for your body. Over time, this personalized approach will help you **gain more confidence and control over diabetes management**, leading to a healthier, more balanced life.

Tips for Successful Journaling

To get the most out of your Personalized Diabetes Journal, try these helpful strategies:

- **Be Consistent**: Choose a regular time each day to jot down your entries—morning reflections or evening recaps work well.

- **Use Short Notes**: You don't have to write long paragraphs. Bullet points or quick phrases are enough to capture key information.

- **Review Weekly**: Set aside time once a week to look back at your entries. Look for trends or patterns, and adjust your goals accordingly.

- **Celebrate Small Wins**: Recognize and reward your progress—whether it's drinking more water, walking consistently, or keeping blood sugar in range.

This small daily habit can lead to lasting improvements in your health, energy, and confidence.

DAILY HEALTH JOURNAL
FOR DIABETICS

Date: _____

Day of the Week: _____

Daily Goal: _____

Start of the Day: Health Check

Wake-up time: _____
Fasting Blood Glucose: _____
Blood Pressure: _____ / _____
Heart Rate (Pulse): _____
Water Intake (planned): _____
Body Temperature (if needed): _____
Sleep Quality: Good / Average / Poor
🏃 Morning Physical Activity (if any):
_____

End of the Day: Health Check

Planned Sleep Time: _____
Blood Glucose Before Bed: _____
Blood Pressure: _____ / _____
Heart Rate (Pulse): _____
Water Intake (fact): _____
Body Temperature (if needed): _____
Physical Activity During the Day:
_____
Overall Well-Being: Good / Average / Poor

Meals & Nutrition

Breakfast
Time: _____
Foods & Portions: _____
_____
✓ *Carbohydrates:* _____

Lunch
Time: _____
Foods & Portions: _____
_____
✓ *Carbohydrates:* _____

Dinner
Time: _____
Foods & Portions: _____
_____
✓ *Carbohydrates:* _____

Snacks & Dessert
Time: _____
Foods & Portions: _____
_____
✓ *Carbohydrates:* _____

Drinks
Time: _____
Foods & Portions: _____
_____
✓ *Carbohydrates:* _____

SELF-MONITORING TABLE

Time of Day	Blood Glucose (mmol/L) 2 hours after eating	Blood Pressure (mmHg)	Medication	Water Intake (Glasses)	Food quality
Morning (Fasting)		____/____	✔ / ✘		
Before Lunch		____/____	✔ / ✘		
After Lunch		____/____	✔ / ✘		
Before Dinner		____/____	✔ / ✘		
Before Bed		____/____	✔ / ✘		

■ DAILY REVIEW

✔ Overall Well-Being:
✔ Any Blood Sugar Spikes? <u>Yes / No</u>
✔ Emotional State:
✔ Was Physical Activity Completed? <u>Yes / No</u>
✔ What Went Well Today: _____
✔ What to Improve Tomorrow: _____

_____

_____
My Goal for Tomorrow: _____

_____

_____
Ketone Check (if needed): _____

NOTES

▪ _____
▪ _____
▪ _____

Health is a daily choice! Keep moving forward!

Monthly №__ Health Log

FOR DIABETICS

Profile Information

- Name: _____
- Date: _____
- Age: _____
- Weight start: ___ kg/lbs; Weight end: ___ kg/lbs
- Height: _____ cm/inches

Monthly Overview

Weeks	Fasting Blood Glucose (mmol/L)	Blood Pressure (mmHg)	♥ Heart Rate (Pulse)	Ketone Check	Meal Quality Avg (1-10)	Physical Activity (Minutes)	Notes
Week 1							
Week 2							
Week 3							
Week 4							

Monthly Summary:

Average Fasting Blood Glucose: _____
Average Blood Glucose Before Bed: _____
Overall Well-Being:
Total Physical Activity (Minutes): _____
Total Water Intake (Glasses): _____
What Went Well This Month: _____
_____
Areas for Improvement: _____
_____

My Goal for Next Month:

_____
_____
_____
_____
_____
_____
_____
_____
_____

Overall Well-Being:

Additional Notes & Medications: _____
_____
_____

Remember: Progress is a journey, keep making small positive steps each day!

Monthly Reflection: Assess, Adjust, and Thrive

As each month comes to a close, take a moment to reflect on your journey toward better diabetes management. By tracking patterns, identifying successes, and making necessary adjustments, you can refine your approach to maintaining balanced blood sugar levels and overall well-being. Use the prompts below to guide your reflection:

Reviewing Your Progress

- **Blood Sugar Balance:** Which foods contributed most to stabilizing your glucose levels?
- **Unexpected Fluctuations:** Did you experience any sudden spikes or drops? Can you identify possible triggers?
- **Activity & Energy:** How did your daily movement or exercise routine influence your energy and glucose levels?
- **Sleep & Emotional Well-Being:** Have you noticed improvements in your sleep quality, stress levels, or overall mood?
- **Medications & Habits:** Were there any changes in your medication, routine, or lifestyle that impacted your results?

📌 **Reflection Notes:** (Jot down key insights and observations from this month.)

Goal Setting for Lasting Success

Progress is built on consistent, achievable steps. Establish clear goals to keep yourself on track:

✔️ **Short-Term Goals (Daily/Weekly)**
Example: *"Incorporate more fiber-rich foods into my breakfasts to promote steady blood sugar levels."*

✔️ **Medium-Term Goals (1-2 Months)**
Example: *"Commit to exercising at least four times a week and monitor my glucose levels before and after workouts."*

✔️ **Long-Term Goals (3+ Months)**
Example: *"Maintain stable blood sugar levels and work toward improving my A1C results."*

Your Commitment to Better Health

By actively engaging in this monthly reflection, you're taking charge of your health and well-being. Small, mindful adjustments lead to long-term success. Stay consistent, celebrate progress, and keep moving forward—one step at a time.

APPENDIX MEASUREMENT CONVERSION CHART

VOLUME EQUIVALENTS (DRY)

US STANDARD	METRIC (APPROXIMATE)
1/8 teaspoon	0.5 mL
1/4 teaspoon	1 mL
1/2 teaspoon	2 mL
3/4 teaspoon	4 mL
1 teaspoon	5 mL
1 tablespoon	15 mL
1/4 cup	59 mL
1/2 cup	118 mL
3/4 cup	177 mL
1 cup	235 mL
2 cups	475 mL
3 cups	700 mL
4 cups	1 L

WEIGHT EQUIVALENTS

US STANDARD	METRIC (APPROXIMATE)
1 ounce	28 g
2 ounces	57 g
5 ounces	142 g
10 ounces	284 g
15 ounces	425 g
16 ounces	455 g
(1 pound)	680 g
1.5 pounds	907 g

VOLUME EQUIVALENTS (LIQUID)

US STANDARD	US STANDARD (OUNCES)	METRIC (APPROXIMATE)
2 tablespoons	1 fl.oz.	30 mL
1/4 cup	2 fl.oz.	60 mL
1/2 cup	4 fl.oz.	120 mL
1 cup	8 fl.oz.	240 mL
1 1/2 cup	12 fl.oz.	355 mL
2 cups or 1 pint	16 fl.oz.	475 mL
4 cups or 1 quart	32 fl.oz.	1 L
1 gallon	128 fl.oz.	4 L

TEMPERATURES EQUIVALENTS

FAHRENHEIT(F)	CELSIUS(C) (APPROXIMATE)
225 °F	107 °C
250 °F	120 °C
275 °F	135 °C
300 °F	150 °C
325 °F	160 °C
350 °F	180 °C
375 °F	190 °C
400 °F	205 °C
425 °F	220 °C
450 °F	235 °C
475 °F	245 °C
500 °F	260 °C

Meet the Author – Andrew Moore

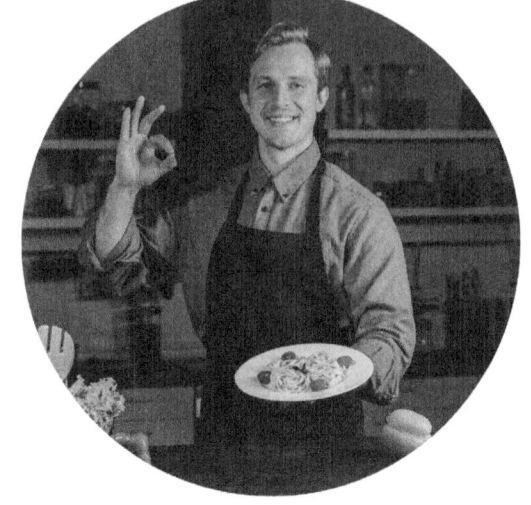

Scan the QR code to follow Andrew on Amazon!

Get notified about:

✔ New cookbooks

✔ Special discounts

✔ Bonus healthy recipes

Andrew Moore is a cookbook author and food enthusiast. He helps thousands of readers discover quick and healthy recipes for everyday life.

Based in California,
Author of 5+ bestselling cookbooks
Passionate about healthy & clean eating

👉 **Follow Andrew on Amazon and never miss a new release or tip!**

Printed in Dunstable, United Kingdom